Instructor's Manual to Accompany

Introduction to Critical Care Nursing

SECOND EDITION

Barbara A. Brown, RN, MN, CCRN
Professor
Community College Allegheny County
Pittsburgh, Pennsylvania

Cheryl Graham-Eason, RN, MEd, MS, CS, CRRN
Professor
Community College Allegheny County
Pittsburgh, Pennsylvania

W.B. Saunders Company
A Division of Harcourt Brace & Company
Philadelphia   London   Toronto   Montreal   Sydney   Tokyo

W. B. SAUNDERS COMPANY

A Division of Harcourt Brace & Company

The Curtis Center
Independence Square West
Philadelphia, Pennsylvania 19106

Instructor's Manual to Accompany
INTRODUCTION TO
CRITICAL CARE NURSING, 2nd Edition   ISBN 0–7216–6219–6

Printed in the United States of America

Last digit is the print number: 9   8   7   6   5   4   3   2   1

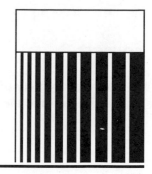

Preface

The authors of this manual have used Hartshorn, Lamborn, and Sole's *Introduction to Critical Care Nursing* to teach nursing students in clinical and classroom settings. Over time, it has become evident that student nurses need guidance in how to utilize this text and apply its contents in the limited time available. Therefore, this first manual has been developed. The elements were designed to be used as follows:

TERMINOLOGY

- To focus students' learning
- To provide short definitions to guide students

Note: The key terms are listed in each chapter and can be copied for students with the outlines and case studies, or the master list with definitions can be copied.

CHAPTER OUTLINES

- To copy as student handouts to facilitate note taking
- To assist with structuring class meetings and curriculum

CHAPTER CASE STUDIES

- To facilitate students' ability to think critically about the application of theory in practice
- To distribute to students as assignments or work sheets
- To use as overheads in class

Note: One set of case studies has blanks for students to complete or for the instructor to show as an overhead and complete with the class. Or the instructor may choose to copy the completed case studies to display in the classroom as the students review their work.

MULTIPLE CHOICE QUESTIONS

- To provide questions directly from the text to assess students' understanding of the reading

Note: Test questions are often difficult to create, so most instructors use a combination of self authored questions and multiple test banks. The authors believe it is helpful to offer a few questions directly from the book to encourage students to recognize the importance of assigned readings.

SOURCES:

- To offer a variety of videos and other materials as an adjunct to the text

The authors can be contacted for comments on this instructor manual via e-mail:

BBrown@CCAC.edu

CGraham@CCAC.edu

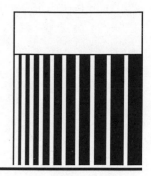

Acknowledgments

We would like to thank Deidre Jarvis for her excellent typing and efficiency in meeting deadlines; we have asked for things yesterday and somehow she has managed to give them to us.

We also give thanks to our parents and our "Jims" who, over time, have seen us do "just one more project."

And to Eric Linn, our teaching assistant, who sat at the computer looking for videos through as many Searches as are available "out there."

Contents

Overview of Critical Care Nursing

Students and new graduates tend to focus on learning the highly technological skills required in critical care settings. This chapter offers the learner an overview of the professional standards or framework for providing these skills. New practitioners should be encouraged to recognize the difference among structure, process, and outcome standards; and discuss who sets the profession's standards and the need for certification. The instructor can utilize this chapter as a point of reference for a critical care course, emphasizing that critically ill patients are found in multiple settings, that both patient and family are experiencing the situation, and that critical care nursing is itself evolving in its scope.

Chapter 2

Individual and Family Response to the Critical Care Experience

TERMINOLOGY

- Anger
- Burnout
- Circadian rhythm
- Desynchronization
- Exacerbate
- ICU syndrome
- Infradian rhythms

- Physical stress
- Powerlessness
- Psychological stress
- Sensory deprivation
- Sensory overload
- Synchronizers
- Ultradian rhythms

OUTLINE

I. Introduction: Interrelationships between psychological and physiological stressors

II. The patient
    A. Alteration in circadian rhythms

    B. Powerlessness

        1. Factors

            a. Environment

            b. Activities of daily living

        c. Timing of family visits/treatment

        d. Lack of knowledge

        2. Behaviors

        3. Nursing interventions

    C. Anger

        1. Factors

        2. Behaviors

D. ICU syndrome

  1. Definition

  2. Factors

    a. Environment

    b. Sleep deprivation

    c. Sensory overload

  3. Goals

E. Individualized patient responses

III. Families and significant others
  A. Family assessment

    1. Family structure

    2. Family functioning

  B. Family stressors and needs

    1. Critical care experience

    2. Need for information

    3. Need for reassurance

    4. Personal needs

  C. Family responses

    1. Fear and anxiety

    2. Dysfunctional families

  D. Interventions

    1. Specific interventions

  2. Adequate education

  3. Additional strategies

    a. Identify nurse's role

    b. Recognize family's usual role

    c. Facilitate family's participation

    d. Explain patient's behaviors (e.g., confusion)

    e. Individualize visiting hours

    f. Educate nurses on common family needs

    g. Explain crisis situation to families

IV. The nurse
  A. Stressors

    1. Shift work

    2. Death of patients

    3. Rapid decision making

    4. Work environment exposures

  B. Burnout

    1. Definition

    2. Symptoms

    3. Prevention

  C. Strategies for job satisfaction

    1. New graduate

    2. Continuing education

MULTIPLE CHOICE

1. An understanding of physical status changes would include which of the following in the nurse's thinking?
   A. All physical status changes relate to obvious physiological changes.
   B. Physical status changes can relate to psychological or environmental stressors.
   C. Physical status changes always develop into ICU syndrome.
   D. Physical status changes relate to physical stressors of critical illness.

Correct answer: B

Rationale: Changes in physical status can be related to the psychological or environment stressors of being in ICU as well as the physical stressors of critical illness.

2. One patient goal that the nurse includes in her care is to:
   A. help the patient maintain circadian synchrony
   B. synchronize ultradian and infradian rhythms
   C. help the patient to desynchronize the ICU environment
   D. help the patient gain control of body rhythms

Correct answer: A

Rationale: The goal is to maintain circadian synchrony.

3. What are common behaviors of a patient who is experiencing powerlessness?
   A. withdrawal and resignation
   B. argumentativeness and sarcasm
   C. hallucinations and paranoia
   D. weeping and thrashing

Correct answer: A

Rationale: Common behaviors include withdrawal and resignation as well as fatalism, lack of decision making ability, aggression, and anger.

4. The nurse would suspect which of the following patients to be at high risk for feelings of powerlessness?
   A. business executives
   B. student nurses
   C. adolescents
   D. young mothers

Correct answer: A

Rationale: Persons who are normally in positions of power or control in their daily lives are more at risk for feelings of powerlessness.

5. Why do patients sometimes not demonstrate or externalize their anger?
   A. They are dependent on others.
   B. Anger is not socially acceptable.
   C. Stoicism is important to them.
   D. Externalizing anger results in physiological consequences.

Correct answer: A

Rationale: Fear of angering those they depend on is the primary reason many patients suppress their anger.

6. The ICU syndrome is most common in patients who have had _____.
   A. renal transplants
   B. cardiotomy surgeries
   C. cranial surgeries
   D. orthopedic surgeries

Correct answer: B

Rationale: Studies have shown that patients with cardiac valve surgeries are more likely to experience this syndrome.

7. The nurse in critical care environments must often assist the family as well as the patient. What is the first part of family assessment?
   A. family functioning
   B. previous family exposure to critical care
   C. existing family problems
   D. family structure

Correct answer: D

Rationale: Assessment of family structure is essential before specific interventions can be designed.

8. Multiple studies have identified the needs of families of the critically ill. What is generally the highest priority of these families?
   A. reassurance
   B. information
   C. personal needs
   D. financial needs

Correct answer: B

Rationale: These studies have revealed that information is a top priority.

9. Some strategies for helping families include:
   A. encouraging family members to take notes
   B. personalizing communication
   C. provision of consistent nurses
   D. all of the above

Correct answer: D

Rationale: These strategies, as well as participating in care and reading educational pamphlets, are valued highly by family members of critically ill patients.

10. Nurses also experience stress in the critical care unit even though working in this area is rewarding. Factors that can cause stress include shift work, death of patients, and the need to make rapid decisions. What can nurses do to prevent burnout?
    A. Set realistic goals.
    B. See work as a career not a job.
    C. Seek support to maintain self-esteem.
    D. all of the above

Correct answer: D

Rationale: All of these should be seriously considered in dealing with stress in ICU.

CASE STUDIES

CASE STUDY #1

Nurses who work in critical care are at high risk for burnout. Discuss some of the factors that could cause this.

> Shift work, in which circadian rhythm is disrupted; working when family is free and vice versa; health factors; family demands; environmental factors such as sensory overload, peer conflicts, floating, lack of input in unit administrative decisions; seeing patients die, especially seeing them die without dignity.

What should nurses do to help prevent this phenomenon?

> Recognize stress overload, develop stress reduction methods, attempt to surround self with optimistic coworkers, praise, focus on the positive, develop hobbies and time management skills.

CASE STUDY #2

Families of critically ill patients also experience emotional difficulties. Identify these.

> Fear and anxiety, especially fear of death of loved one; lack of understanding of equipment; fear of temporary changes in family roles; financial concerns; concerns about already existing family problems.

What can the nurse do for these families?

> Develop methods of communication such as "telefamily," provide consistent nurses to work with patients, develop support groups and educational brochures, personalize communication by calling family members by their names, identify self as the nurse responsible for their loved one, and most importantly establish a method of keeping family members informed of changes in the patient's status and of the purpose of equipment

Chapter 2 Case Studies

CASE STUDY #1

Nurses who work in critical care are at high risk for burnout. Discuss some of the factors that could cause this.

What should nurses do to help prevent this phenomenon?

CASE STUDY #2

Families of critically ill patients also experience emotional difficulties. Identify these. What can the nurse do for these families?

Symptoms of Burnout

PHYSIOLOGICAL	BEHAVIORAL	EMOTIONAL
Fatigue	Increased absenteeism	Withdrawal from work and family
Headaches	Impatience	Depression
Cold, clammy hands	Alcohol and drug addiction	Irritability
Nausea/vomiting	Rigidity	Anger
Diarrhea	Accident proneness	Indifference
Muscle tension	Low productivity	Detachment
Elevated blood pressure	Overactivity	Hostility
Excessive urination	Compulsive eating	Avoidance
Profuse sweating	Inability to eat	Pessimism
Increased respiration	Forgetfulness	Crying
Increased pulse rate	Restlessness	Anxiety
	Sleeplessness	Frustration
	Loss of interest	

Examples of Biological Rhythms

CIRCADIAN RHYTHMS

- Sleep/wakefulness
- Body temperature
- Blood pressure
- Urine flow

ULTRADIAN RHYTHMS

- REM/NREM sleep
- Sinoatrial node firing
- Nerve action potential

INFRADIAN RHYTHMS

- Menstrual cycle
- Hibernation
- Aging

Common Stressors for ICU Nurses

COMMON STRESSORS

- Intricate, ever-changing technology

- Participating in resuscitation, death, and dying

- Long shifts with considerable physical labor

- Ethical dilemmas

- Compromised socialization due to working shifts and weekends

- Occupational hazards (e.g., infections, radiation)

STRATEGIES FOR STRESS REDUCTION

- Continuous learning, reading, working with mentors

- Debriefing with coworkers after the event

- Good physical health habits (e.g., healthy diet and exercise)

- Consultation with peers, managers, ethicists, or ethics committee

- Creating opportunities for socializing at work and with coworkers on similar work schedules

- Learning and adhering to universal and other safety precautions

Ethical and Legal Issues in Critical Care Nursing

TERMINOLOGY

- Abandonment
- Advance directives
- Beneficence
- Brain Death
- Doctrine of informed consent

- Irreversible coma or persistent vegetative state
- Negligence
  Acts of commission
  Acts of omission
- Nonmaleficence

OUTLINE

E. Selected legal ethical issues

   1. Informed consent

      a. Elements of informed consent

      b. Informed consent of adolescents

      c. Emergency treatment

      d. Emancipated minors

      e. Minor treatment statutes

   2. Withholding or withdrawing life-sustaining treatment

      a. Extraordinary treatment

      b. Withholding or withdrawing life support

         1. *Barber* v. *Superior Court* (1985)

         2. *Cruzan* v. *Director* (1990)

            a. Patient Self determination Act (1990)

            b. Advance directives

   3. Organ tissue transplantation

   4. Care of persons with HIV/AIDS

CASE STUDIES

CASE STUDY #1

Nurses in critical care often care for patients who have illnesses that lead to irreversible coma and subsequently brain death. Some of these patients have indicated prior to their illness a willingness to donate their organs. One such patient has just died, and the nurse and physician are discussing this with the patient's wife. She does not want this wish honored. What legal and ethical issues must be considered?

> The legal ramification of the patient's wish; the patient's competency; the clarity of the patient's wishes; the ethical code of nurses and the nurse's role as advocate, inlcuding the legal interpretation of the advocate as standing in; the wife's response to the sudden loss of a loved one and assisting her to grieve while not losing valuable time in harvesting the organs; and the nurse's need to deal with his or her own beliefs and values regarding life and death.

CASE STUDY #2

A well-known video demonstrates the life of a young man who was severely burned in an explosion. This man is now married with children and is productive at work. He had requested to be allowed to die at the time of the injury and this request was not honored. What are the ramifications for this man and health care providers when someone else (e.g., the patient's mother) makes a decision contrary to the patient's wishes?

> Case law should be discussed, ethical issues regarding self-determination need to be considered, principles of ethical decision making should be reviewed one by one to see how they apply. (The final answer in this case, as in many others, is not always clear.)

Chapter Three Case Studies

CASE STUDY #1

Nurses in critical care often care for patients who have illnesses that lead to irreversible coma and subsequently brain death. Some of these patients have indicated prior to their illness a willingness to donate their organs. One such patient has just died, and the nurse and physician are discussing this with the patient's wife. She does not want this wish honored. What legal and ethical issues must be considered?

CASE STUDY #2

A well-known video dramatizes the life of a young man who was severely burned in an explosion. This man is now married with children and is productive at work. He had requested to be allowed to die at the time of the injury and this request was not honored. What are the ramifications for this man and health care providers when someone else (e.g., the patient's mother) makes a decision contrary to the patient's wishes?

The American Nurses' Association Code of Ethics

1. The nurse provides services with respect for human dignity and the uniqueness of the client unrestricted by considerations of social or economic status, personal attributes, or the nature of health problems.

2. The nurse safeguards the client's right to privacy by judiciously protecting information of a confidential nature.

3. The nurse acts to safeguard the client and the public when health care and safety are affected by the incompetent, unethical, or illegal practices of any person.

4. The nurse assumes responsibility and accountability for individual nursing judgments and actions.

5. The nurse maintains competence in nursing.

6. The nurse exercises informed judgment and uses individual competence and qualifications as criteria in seeking consultation, accepting responsibilities, and delegating nursing activities to others.

7. The nurse participates in acitivites that contribute to the ongoing development of the profession's body of knowledge.

8. The nurse participates in the profession's efforts to implement and improve standards of nursing.

9. The nurse participates in the profession's efforts to establish and maintain conditions of employment conducive to high quality nursing care.

10. The nurse participates in the profession's effort to protect the public from misinformation and misrepresentation and to maintain the integrity of nursing.

11. The nurse collaborates with members of the health professions and other citizens in promoting community and national efforts to meet the health needs of the public.

Tests Used to Determine Brain Death

1.   Cessation of spontaneous respiration

2.   Cessation of spontaneous heartbeat

3.   Cessation of brain function, including absence of all function of the brainstem and cerebral hemispheres; verified by the following findings in the absence of hypothermia or drug-induced states:

   —   no response on neurological examination

   —   isoelectric electroencephalogram (EEG)

   —   absence of cerebral blood flow

(These tests are formalized criteria for brain death used by various institutions and groups, such as the Harvard Medical School Ad Hoc Committee and the National Institute of Health Collaborative Study of Cerebral Survival. No absolute criteria exist for determining brain death.)

Chapter 4

Dysrhythmia Interpretation

TERMINOLOGY

- Aberrant conduction
- Antidysrhythmic
- Asynchronous mode
- Asystole
- Atrial kick
- Atrioventricular (AV) block
- AV dissociation
- Beta blockers
- Bipolar
- Bradycardia
- Calcium channel blocker
- Capture
- Cardiac glycoside
- Demand mode
- Depolarization
- Diastole
- Dromotropy
- Dysrhythmia
- Ectopic
- Electrocardiography
- Electrophysiology
- Fibrillation
- Idioventricular rhythm

- Intercostal
- Junctional/nodal rhythm
- Milliamperes
- Multifocal
- P wave
- Pacemaker
- Parasympathetic nervous system (PNS)
- Paroxysmal
- QRS complex
- Repolarization
- Sense (sensitivity)
- Sinus rhythm
- Sympathetic nervous system (SNS)
- Systole
- T wave
- Tachycardia
- Threshold
- Transthoracic
- Transvenous
- Vagal maneuvers
- Vagolytic
- Valsalva's maneuver

OUTLINE

I. Electrocardiography
    A. Definition

    B. Electrocardiogram

II. Basic electrophysiology
     A. Automaticity

     B. Blood flow

     C. Nervous supply

III. Cardiac cycle
      A. Electrical activity

      1. Depolarization

      2. Repolarization

      B. Mechanical activity

      1. Diastole

      2. Systole

      C. Cardiac action potential

      1. Electrolyte movement

      a. Resting membrane potential

      1. Charge

      2. Millivolts

      b. Depolarization

      1. Sodium

      2. Potassium

      c. Repolarization

D. Relationship between electrical activity and muscular contraction

   1. Electrocardiogram (ECG) tracing

   2. Clinical signs of cardiac systole

   3. Death

      a. ECG tracing

      b. Automaticity

      c. Pulseless electrical activity (PEA)

IV. Normal conduction pathway
     A. Special cardiac cells—impulse generation

     B. SA node

     C. Internodal pathways

     D. Atria—characteristics

     E. Atrial depolarization

        1. Atrial systole/atrial kick

     F. Atrioventricular (AV) node

        1. Conduction pathway

        2. Pacemaker

     G. Ventricular conduction

        1. Bundle of His

        2. Bundle branches

           a. Right bundle branch

b. Left bundle branch

3. Purkinje fibers

V. 12-lead EKG
   A. Standard limb leads

   1. Bipolar

   2. Lead I

   3. Lead II

   4. Lead III

   B. Augmented limb leads

   1. Unipolar

   2. aVR

   3. aVL

   4. aVF

   C. Precordial leads

   1. Landmarks

   2. Use

   D. Monitoring

   1. Timing

   2. Lead placement

   3. Preferred leads for clinical setting

      a. Lead II

      b. V1

c. MCL1

4. 12-lead ECG

VI. Analyzing ECG tracing
    A. ECG paper

    1. Measure time

       a. Seconds

       b. Value

    2. Measure height/amplitude

       a. Millimeter

       b. Voltage

    B. Waveforms and intervals

    1. Isoelectric line

    2. P Wave

       a. Atrial depolarization

       b. Configuration

       c. Amplitude

       d. Indicators

    3. PR interval

       a. Measurement

       b. Description of normal

       c. Abnormal PRs

    4. QRS

a. Description of normal

   1. Q wave

   2. R wave

   3. S wave

b. QRS interval

   1. Measurement

5. T wave

  a. Identification

  b. Description

  c. Meaning of changes in T wave

6. ST segment

  a. Description

  b. QT intervals

    1. Measurement

    2. Description of normal

7. U wave

  a. Description

  b. Meaning

C. Systematic interpretation of dysrhythmias

  1. Rhythmicity

    a. Definition

    b. Atrial rhythmicity

c. Ventricular rhythmicity

d. Use of calipers

e. Paper and pencil

f. Irregular rhythms

2. Rate

  a. Definition

  b. Assessment

    1. Rule of 1500

    2. Rule of 10

  c. Monitor display rate

3. Waveform configuration and location

  a. Configuration

    1. Definition

    2. Description of normal

    3. Importance

  b. Location

    1. Importance

    2. Normal

4. Assessment of intervals

VIII. Basic dysrhythmias
  A. Definitions

    1. Dysrhythmia

2. Arrhythmia

B. Interpreting

  1. Critical criteria

  2. Hemodynamics

C. Normal sinus rhythm

  1. Critical criteria

    a. P wave

    b. Rates

    c. Rhythm

    d. Intervals

    e. Hemodynamics

D. Sinus bradycardia

  1. Definition

  2. Causative processes

    a. Vagal stimulation

    b. Drug effects

    c. SA node ischemia

    d. Effects of hypoxia

    e. As a normal finding

    f. Increased ICP

  3. Critical criteria

  4. Hemodynamics

E. Sinus tachycardia

  1. Definition

  2. Causative processes

    a. Exercise

    b. Stimulants

    c. Increased body temperature

    d. Altered fluid status

  3. Critical criteria

  4. Hemodynamics

F. Sinus dysrhythmia

  1. Definition

  2. Physiology

  3. Critical criteria

  4. Hemodynamics

G. Sinus arrest/sinus exit block

  1. Definition

  2. ECG description

  3. Causes

    a. Enhanced vagal tone

    b. CAD

    c. Drugs

  4. Critical criteria

5. Hemodynamics

H. Atrial dysrhythmias

   1. Processes that cause increased automaticity

      a. Stress

      b. Electrolyte imbalances

      c. Hypoxia

      d. Atrial injury

      e. Digitalis toxicity

      f. Hypothermia

      g. Hyperthyroidism

      h. Alcohol intoxication

      i. Pericarditis

   2. Premature atrial contractions

      a. Description

      b. Critical criteria

      c. Blocked premature atrial contraction

         1. Critical criteria

      d. Hemodynamics

   3. Wandering atrial pacemaker (WAP)

      a. Description

      b. Critical criteria

      c. Hemodynamics

   4. Multifocal atrial tachycardia

      a. Description

      b. Critical criteria

      c. Hemodynamics

   5. Paroxysmal atrial tachycardia

      a. Description

      b. Critical criteria

      c. Hemodynamics

   6. Atrial flutter

      a. Description

      b. Critical criteria

      c. Hemodynamics

   7. Atrial fibrillation

      a. Description

         1. Ashman's beats

         2. Mural thrombi

      b. Critical criteria

      c. Hemodynamics

I. AV dysrhythmias

   1. Description

   2. Primary causes

      a. Ectopic

b. Escape

3. P wave changes

   a. Absent

   b. Inverted

   c. After QRS

4. PR interval changes

5. Junctional/nodal rhythm

   a. Critical criteria

   b. Hemodynamics

6. Junctional tachycardia/accelerated nodal rhythm

   a. Description

   b. Critical criteria

   c. Hemodynamics

7. Premature junctional contractions

   a. Description

      1. Noncompensatory

      2. Compensatory

   b. Critical criteria

   c. Hemodynamics

J. Ventricular dysrhythmias

1. Description

   a. Ectopic

b. Escape

2. Causes

   a. Myocardial ischemia, injury, and infarction

   b. Hypokalemia

   c. Hypomagnesemia

   d. Hypoxia

   e. Acid-base imbalance

3. Premature ventricular contractions

   a. Description

      1. Patterns

      2. Vulnerable period

      3. Occurrence

   b. Critical criteria

   c. Hemodynamics

4. Ventricular tachycardia

   a. Description

   b. Critical criteria

   c. Hemodynamics

5. Ventricular fibrillation

   a. Description

      1. Coarse

      2. Fine

b. Critical criteria

c. Hemodynamics

6. Idioventricular rhythm

  a. Description

  b. Critical criteria

  c. Hemodynamics

7. Accelerated idioventricular rhythm

  a. Description

  b. Critical criteria

  c. Hemodynamics

8. Ventricular standstill

  a. Description

  b. Critical criteria

    1. Coarse

    2. Fine

  c. Hemodynamics

K. AV blocks

1. Description

2. Causes

  a. CAD

  b. Infectious/inflammatory processes

  c. Vagal tone

d. Drugs

3. Types of blocks

  a. First degree

    1. Critical criteria

    2. Hemodynamics

  b. Second degree

    1. Description

    2. Critical criteria

    3. Hemodynamics

  c. Second degree type II: Mobitz II

    1. Description

    2. Critical criteria

    3. Hemodynamics

  d. Third degree

    1. Description

    2. AV dissociation

    3. Backup pacemakers

    4. ECG waveforms

    5. Critical criteria

    6. Hemodynamics

IX. Interventions
  A. Advanced cardiac life support (ACLS)

B. Tachycardias

  1. Premature beats

    a. Treatment

    b. Symptoms

  2. Differentiating between supraventricular tachycardia (SVT) and ventricular tachycardia (VT)

    a. Description

    b. Rapid-rate dysrhythmias

    c. Symptoms

    d. Treatment

  3. Mediating effects of the nervous system

    a. Sympathetic nervous system

    b. Relaxation techniques

    c. Pain and anxiety relief

    d. Vagal maneuvers

      1. Carotid massage

      2. Valsalva's maneuver

  4. Intervening with cardiac drugs

    a. Antidysrhythmics

      1. Adenosine

      2. Lidocaine

    b. Beta blockers

      1. SNS

      2. Setting MI

      3. Effects

    c. Calcium channel blockers

      1. Use

      2. Diltiazem

      3. Verapamil

    d. Cardiac glycosides

      1. Digoxin, digitoxin

      2. Digitalized

      3. Effects

      4. Toxicity

  5. Intervening with electrical energy

    a. Situations when used

    b. Types of electrical treatment modalities

      1. Synchronized cardioversion

        a. Energy

        b. Delivery

        c. Equipment

        d. Effects

      2. Defibrillation

      3. Implantable cardioverter-defibrillator

a. Uses

b. Description

c. Programmed

d. Patient activity

4. Radio frequency ablation

a. Uses

b. Description

C. Bradycardia

1. Rhythms treated

2. Signs and symptoms

3. Suppression of parasympathetic system

a. Vagus nerve/vagal tone

b. Nausea and vomiting

c. Hypoxia

4. Drugs

a. Atropine

b. Isoproterenol

c. Dopamine

d. Epinephrine

e. Drug effects

5. Pacemakers

a. Indications

b. Temporary

1. Generators

2. External pacemaking

a. Description

b. Modes

c. Use as a bridge

3. Transvenous pacemaking

a. Description

b. Bipolar

c. AV sequential

d. Pacing

i. Pacer spike

ii. Wave configuration

iii. Capture

iv. Threshold

v. Rate

vi. Sensitivity

vii. Securing generator

viii. Electrical safety

e. Troubleshooting

i. Failure to capture

ii. Failure to sense

D. Pulseless rhythms

    1. Ventricular fibrillation/ventricular tachycardia without a pulse

        a. Life threatening

        b. Diagnosing

        c. Treatment

           1. CPR

           2. Defibrillation

           3. Drugs

    2. Asystole

        a. Prognosis

        b. Treatment

MULTIPLE CHOICE

---

1. The ECG tracing provides evidence of the patient's
   A. pulse
   B. blood pressure
   C. heart rate
   D. temperature

Correct answer: C

Rationale: ECG tracing shows that the cardiac muscles are generating electrical activity.

2. Depolarization begins when _____ ions move into the cardiac cell.
   A. chloride
   B. magnesium
   C. potassium
   D. sodium

Correct answer: D

Rationale: Sodium ions move into the cardiac cell while potassium ions move out of the cell.

3. A patient was pronounced dead but there was still an ECG tracing present. This happens because of the myocardial property of
   A. automaticity
   B. conductivity
   C. contractility
   D. refractoriness

Correct answer: A

Rationale: Automaticity is the heart's ability to initiate its own electrical impulses despite lack of blood and nerve supply.

4. Depolarization precedes
   A. diastole
   B. systole
   C. resting potential
   D. action potential

Correct answer: B

Rationale: Electrical stimulation along the conduction pathways precede myocardial contraction.

5. Atrial kick is provided by atrial contraction at the end of diastole. It supplies a 30% increase in
   A. cardiac output
   B. left ventricular end diastolic volume
   C. left atrial end diastolic volume
   D. cardiac index

Correct answer: B

Rationale: Atrial kick contributes an approximate 30% increase in blood sent to the ventricles.

6. Each small block on ECG paper measures time equal to
   A. 2.0 milliseconds
   B. 0.20 seconds
   C. 4.0 milliseconds
   D. 0.04 seconds

Correct answer: D

Rationale: Each small box is equal to 0.04 seconds or 40.0 milliseconds.

7. If a ventricular rhythm is regular
   A. each P wave is equidistant from the next R
   B. each R wave is equidistant from the next R
   C. each R wave is equidistant from the next T
   D. each P wave is equidistant from the next P

Correct answer: B

Rationale: When an atrial rhythm is regular, each P wave is equidistant from the next P wave; if the ventricular rhythm is regular, each R wave is equidistant from the next R wave.

8. You are calculating the rate for a regular rhythm. There are 21 small boxes before each R wave. The rate is
   A. 94
   B. 85
   C. 50
   D. 71

Correct answer: D

Rationale: Use the rule of 1500:

$$\frac{1500}{21} = 71 \text{ beats/minute}$$

9. The optimal rhythm for maintaining hemodynamic stability is
   A. SB
   B. AF
   C. SR
   D. AT

Correct answer: C

Rationale: SR is the optimal rhythm for maintaining an adequate CO and BP.

10. The hemodynamic effects of tachyarrhythmia may be caused in part by
    A. increased atrial kick
    B. decreased conductivity
    C. decreased diastolic filling time
    D. increased automaticity

Correct answer: C

Rationale: Tachycardia leads to decreased ventricular filling time which causes decreased ventricular volume in systole which decreases cardiac output and blood pressure.

11. A person who has _____ is predisposed to atrial arrhythmias.
    A. hypothyroidism
    B. alcohol withdrawal
    C. hyperthermia
    D. digitalis toxicity

Correct answer: D

Rationale: Digitalis in toxic doses can be stimulating to the myocardium, particularly the atria.

12. A wandering atrial pacemaker (WAP) is seen most often in patients with
    A. COPD
    B. CAD
    C. CVAH
    D. CPR

Correct answer: A

Rationale: WAP is often seen in COPD patients secondary to hypoxia.

13. The sawtooth waveform of atrial flutter is formed by an irritable focus in the
    A. sinus node
    B. atrial tissue
    C. AV junction
    D. ventricular tissue

Correct answer: B

Rationale: "F" waves of flutter waves arise from a single irritable focus in the atria.

14. Atrial fibrillation is irregularly irregular causing what hemodynamic effect?
    A. decreased LAP
    B. increased LVE DP
    C. loss of atrial kick
    D. loss of ventricular systole

Correct answer: C

Rationale: Loss of atrial kick diminishes effective ventricular filling. This is caused by loss of atrial contraction.

15. A rhythm originating in the AV node with a rate of 98 is called
    A. sinus arrhythmia
    B. junctional rhythm
    C. atrial tachycardia
    D. junctional tachycardia

Correct answer: D

Rationale: Junctional tachycardia includes rates from 60 to 150 beats/minute.

16. Ventricular ectopy may occur with
    A. hypokalemia
    B. hypermagnesemia
    C. hyperoxia
    D. acid-base balance

Correct answer: A

Rationale: Hypokalemia can facilitate the development of ventricular dysrhythmias because potassium plays an important role in the normal depolarization/repolarization process.

17. Idioventricular rhythm means the heart rate is
    A. 100 to 150
    B. 60 to 100
    C. 40 to 60
    D. 15 to 40

Correct answer: D

Rationale: Idioventricular rhythm is an escape rhythm generated by the Purkinje fibers, capable of an intrinsic rate of 15 to 40 beats/minute.

18. The type of AV block which causes the most uncoordinated rhythm is
    A. first degree
    B. Mobitz I
    C. Mobitz II
    D. third degree

Correct answer: D

Rationale: In third degree or complete block, there is no communication between atria and ventricles; each beats at its own rate.

19. If your patient has complete heart block, he or she needs
    A. pacer
    B. digitalis
    C. defibrillation
    D. Lidocaine

Correct answer: A

Rationale: A pacer will stimulate the ventricle to increase heart rate.

20. When a pacer fails to capture, this means
    A. the pacer is transvenous
    B. the pacer is asynchronous
    C. the pacer does not recognize the heart's intrinsic beat
    D. the pacer is not able to cause chamber depolarization

Correct answer: D

Rationale: A pacer spike should produce chamber depolarization either at P or QRS depending upon which chamber is paced.

CASE STUDIES

CASE STUDY #1

Mrs. F. presents in the clinic complaining of fluttering in her chest. She is placed on a cardiac monitor which shows a new onset atrial fibrillation: heart rate $\pm$ 110. She has a history of COPD and CHF and has been taking digoxin and Lasix every day.

1. What is atrial kick?

   Atrial contraction late in diastole contributes extra volume to ventricular filling, increasing ventricular wall stretch to increase strength of contraction in systole.

2. Because Mrs. F. is in atrial fibrillation, she has lost atrial kick. What are the hemodynamic consequences of atrial fibrillation?

   Cardiac output decreases from irregularly irregular rhythm, tachycardia, decreasing diastolic filling time, loss of atrial kick, no atrial contraction.

A cardizem drip is initiated to decrease Mrs. F.'s heart rate. During the admission process, she becomes increasingly congested, wheezy, and restless. ABGs are drawn, which show hypoxemia. She is still in atrial fibrillation and is now having multifocal PVCs.

3. Why is Mrs. F. at risk for digitalis toxicity?

   Her K+ may be low from daily Lasix.

   Her digoxin dose may need to be modified.

4. Describe the pathophysiology of multifocal PVCs and their hemodynamic effects.

   More than one area of irritable ventricular tissue depolarizes prematurely.

   May decrease cardiac output because they are premature and originate on ventricular tissue, (i.e., there is no atrial kick and they follow abnormal conduction pathway).

5. Write two nursing diagnoses for Mrs. F.

   1. Decreased cardiac output related to arrhythmias (atrial fibrillation) and PVCs.

   2. Impaired gas exchange related to ventilation perfusion imbalance (pulmonary congestion, CHF, and COPD).

CASE STUDY #2

82-year-old Mrs. Z. has been frequently falling at home. She sought medical attention when she suffered a broken arm during a fall. In the Emergency Department (ED), her heart rate was in the low 50s. She complained of dizziness and intermittent nausea. Preliminary EKG and lab studies showed evidence of an MI. She was admitted to the Cardiac Care Unit (CCU), where her heart rate dropped to the 40s (sinus bradycardia). An external pacer was applied, (MA-40, HR-70) while arrangements were made for temporary transvenous pacer insertion.

1. What are the hemodynamic consequences of sinus bradycardia (SB)?

    A slow heart rate without an increased stroke volume will decrease cardiac output.

2. What drugs could have been used to increase Mrs. Z.'s heart rate and what are their actions?

    Atropine IVP—vagolytic

    Isuprel drip—sympathomimetic

3. How would you know if the pacer is functioning properly?

    Capture is demonstrated by a pacer spike followed by chamber depolarization; in this case, a QRS complex. The nurse must also check function by palpating the patient's pulse.

4. Write three nursing diagnoses for Mrs. Z.

    1. Decreased cardiac output related to arrhythmias (SB).

    2. Potential for infection related to invasive therapies (IV and pacer insertion).

    3. Pain related to physical injury agents (TCP and pacer insertion).

5. Mrs. Z.'s physician has decided that she needs a permanent pacer. She is refusing, saying that she doesn't want the pacer to keep her alive if it is her time to die. What do you tell her?

    In words she can understand, tell Mrs. Z. that the pacer only causes chamber depolarization and that the myocardium must then contract. If the muscle no longer responds with contraction, the pacer has no life-sustaining effect.

Chapter 4 Case Studies

CASE STUDY #1

Mrs. F. presents in the clinic complaining of fluttering in her chest. She is placed on a cardiac monitor which shows a new onset atrial fibrillation: heart rate $\pm$ 110. She has a history of COPD and CHF and has been taking digoxin and Lasix every day.

1. What is atrial kick?

2. Because Mrs. F. is in atrial fibrillation, she has lost atrial kick. What are the hemodynamic consequences of atrial fibrillation?

A cardizem drip is initiated to decrease Mrs. F.'s heart rate. During the admission process, she becomes increasingly congested, wheezy, and restless. ABGs are drawn, which show hypoxemia. She is still in atrial fibrillation and is now having multifocal PVCs.

3. Why is Mrs. F. at risk for digitalis toxicity?

4. Describe the pathophysiology of multifocal PVCs and their hemodynamic effects.

5. Write two nursing diagnoses for Mrs. F.

Chapter 4 Case Studies

CASE STUDY #2

82-year-old Mrs. Z. has been frequently falling at home. She sought medical attention when she suffered a broken arm during a fall. In the Emergency Department (ED), her heart rate was in the low 50s. She complained of dizziness and intermittent nausea. Preliminary EKG and lab studies showed evidence of an MI. She was admitted to the Cardiac Care Unit (CCU), where her heart rate dropped to the 40s (sinus bradycardia). An external pacer was applied, (MA-40, HR-70) while arrangements were made for temporary transvenous pacer insertion.

1.   What are the hemodynamic consequences of sinus bradycardia (SB)?

2.   What drugs could have been used to increase Mrs. Z.'s heart rate and what are their actions?

3.   How would you know if the pacer is functioning properly?

4.   Write three nursing diagnoses for Mrs. Z.

5.   Mrs. Z.'s physician has decided that she needs a permanent pacer. She is refusing, saying that she doesn't want the pacer to keep her alive if it is her time to die. What do you tell her?

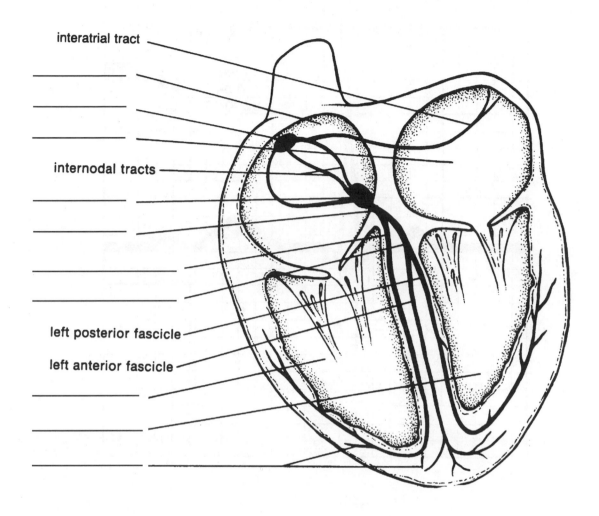

interatrial tract

internodal tracts

left posterior fascicle

left anterior fascicle

DIRECTIONS

1. Label conduction system

2. Draw pacer wires necessary for DDD pacing

Figure 4–2: Normal cardiac conduction pathway. (From Patel, J., McGowan, S., and Moody, L.: Arrythmias: Detection, Treatment, and Cardiac Drugs. Philadelphia, W. B. Saunders, 1989, Fig. 1, p. 2.)

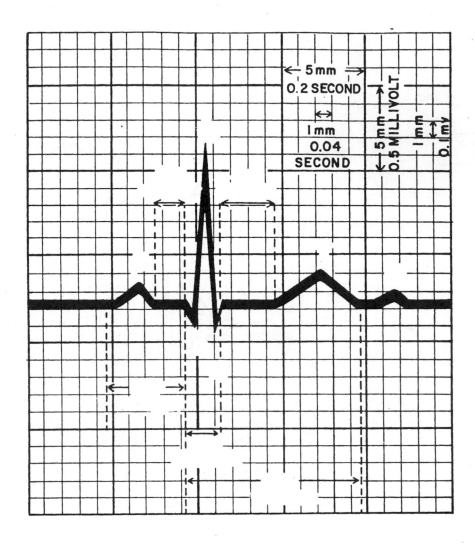

DIRECTIONS

1. Label the horizontal measurements of 1 small box and 1 large box

2. Label waveforms and intervals

Figure 4–9: Normal ECG tracing: Waveforms and intervals. (From Sanderson, R., and Kurth, C.: The Cardiac Patient: A comprehensive Approach. 2nd ed. Philadelphia, W. B. Saunders, 1983, p. 149.)

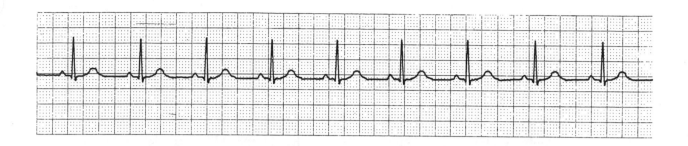

Rate_____   **Rhythm** _____

P wave_____   **PR**_____

QRS_____   **Interpretation** _____

ANSWER

Rate_____71_____   **Rhythm** ___regular_____

P wave___OK_____   **PR**____.16_____

QRS_____.06_____   **Interpretation** __sinus rhythm_____

Figure 4–19: Normal sinus rhythm: Rhythm strip generated by the AA-700 Rhythm Simulator. (Reproduced with permission from Armstrong Medical Industries, Lincolnshire, Illinois, *DataSim*, Fig. 0.)

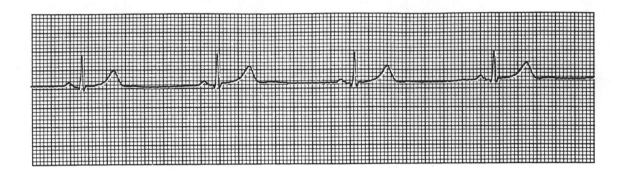

Rate_____   **Rhythm** _____

P wave_____   **PR**_____

QRS_____   **Interpretation** _____

ANSWER

Rate_____41_____   **Rhythm** ___regular_____

P wave___OK_____   **PR**____.16_____

QRS_____.08_____   **Interpretation** __sinus bradycardia_____

Figure 4–20: Sinus bradycardia. (From Davis, D.: ECG Workout: Exercises in Arrhythmia Interpretation. Philadelphia, J. B. Lippincott, 1985, p. 38, sinus bradycardia.)

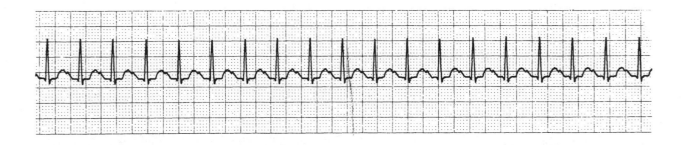

Rate_____   **Rhythm** _____

P wave_____   **PR**_____

QRS_____   **Interpretation** _____

ANSWER

Rate_____136_____   **Rhythm** ____regular_____

P wave____OK_____   **PR**____.16_____

QRS_____.06_____   **Interpretation** __sinus tachycardia_____

Figure 4–21: Sinus tachycardia: Rhythm strip generated by the AA-700 Rhythm Simulator. (Reproduced with permission from Armstrong Medical Industries, Lincolnshire, Illinois, *DataSim*, Fig. 1.)

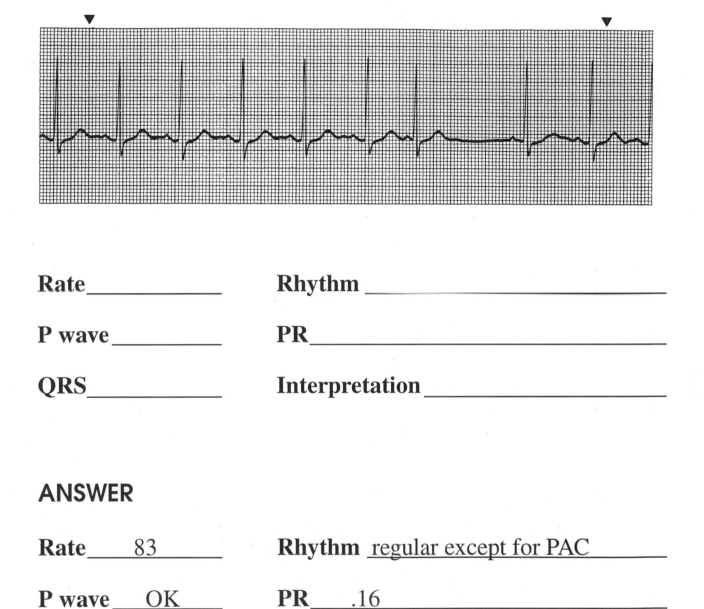

Rate_____ **Rhythm** _____

P wave_____ **PR**_____

QRS_____ **Interpretation** _____

ANSWER

Rate_____83_____ **Rhythm** _regular except for PAC_____

P wave___OK_____ **PR**____.16_____

QRS____.08_____ **Interpretation** _sinus rhythm with____
_premature atrial complex_____

Figure 4–24: Premature atrial contraction. Note noncompensatory pause. (From Huff, J., Doernbach, D., and White, R.: ECG Workout: Exercises in Arrhythmia Interpretation, Philadelphia, J. B. Lippincott, 1985, Fig. 2.5.)

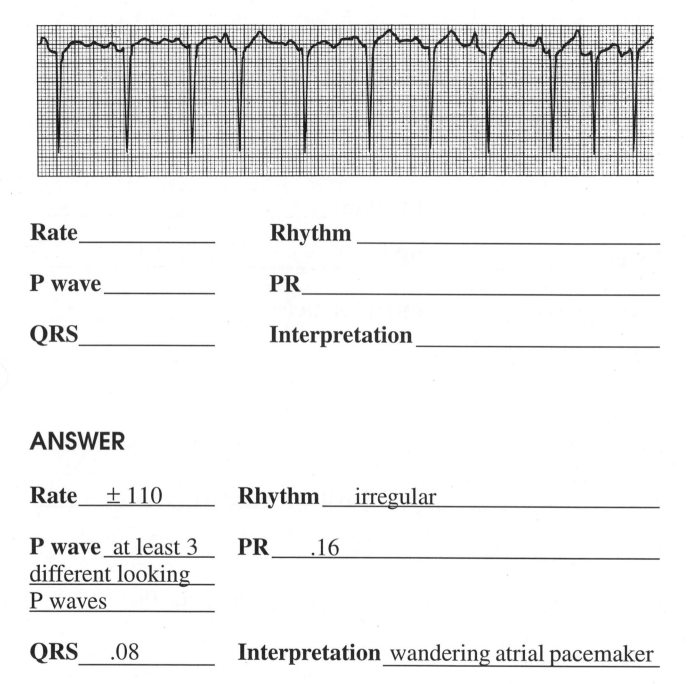

Rate_____ **Rhythm**_____

P wave_____ **PR**_____

QRS_____ **Interpretation**_____

ANSWER

Rate___± 110___ **Rhythm**___irregular_____

P wave _at least 3_ **PR**___.16_____
different looking
P waves

QRS___.08_____ **Interpretation** _wandering atrial pacemaker_

Figure 4–26: Wandering atrial pacemaker. Note the varying P wave morphologies. (From Patel, J., McGowan, S., and Moody, L.: Arrythmias: Detection, Treatment, and Cardiac Drugs. Philadelphia, W. B. Saunders, 1989, Fig. 41.)

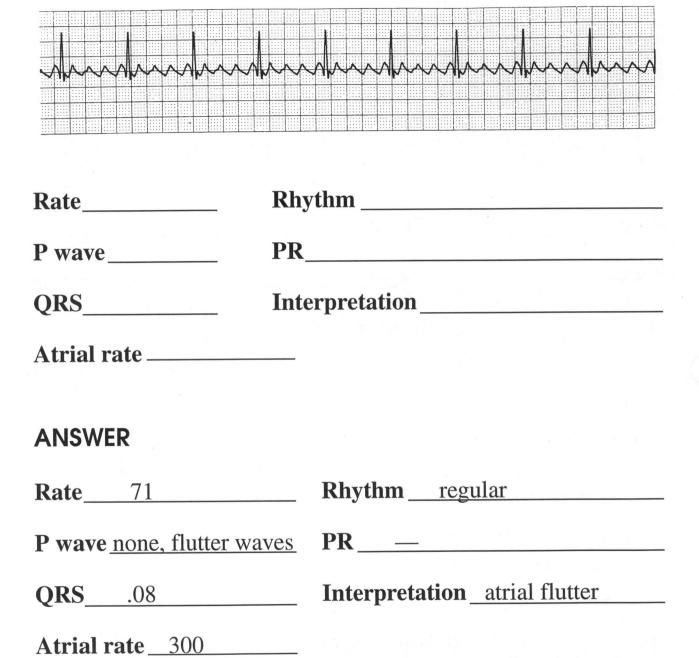

Rate_____ **Rhythm** _____

P wave_____ **PR**_____

QRS_____ **Interpretation** _____

Atrial rate _____

ANSWER

Rate_____71_____ **Rhythm** ___regular_____

P wave <u>none, flutter waves</u> **PR** _____—_____

QRS_____.08_____ **Interpretation** __atrial flutter_____

Atrial rate __300_____

Figure 4–30: Atrial flutter: Note sawtooth configuration and negative orientation of the flutter waves. Rhythm strip generated by the AA-700 Rhythm Simulator. (Reproduced with permission from Armstrong Medical Industries, Lincolnshire, Illinois, *DataSim*, Fig. 4.)

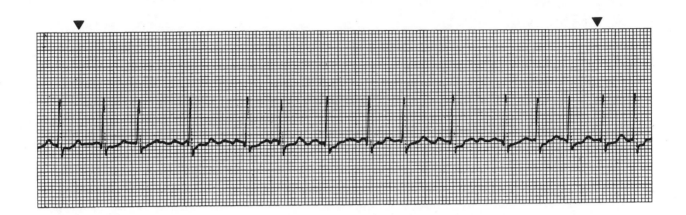

Rate_____   **Rhythm** _____

P wave_____   **PR**_____

QRS_____   **Interpretation** _____

ANSWER

Rate___± 120_____   **Rhythm** ___irregularly irregular_____

P wave____—_____   **PR**____—_____

QRS____.06_____   **Interpretation** _atrial fibrillation_____

Figure 4–34: Atrial fibrillation. (From Huff, J., Doernbach, D., and White, R.: ECG Workout: Exercises in Arrhythmia Interpretation, Philadelphia, J. B. Lippincott, 1985, Fig. 2.50.)

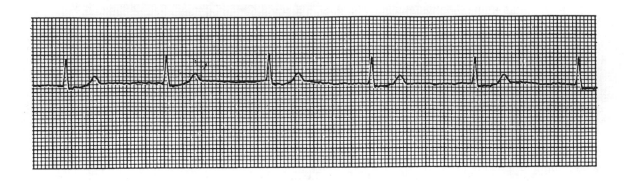

Rate_____   **Rhythm**_____

P wave_____   **PR**_____

QRS_____   **Interpretation**_____

ANSWER

Rate____56____   **Rhythm**____regular_____

P wave___none___   **PR**____—_____

QRS____.08____   **Interpretation**_junctional rhythm_____

Figure 4–35: Nodal/junctional rhythm. Note absence of P waves. (From Davis, D.: How to Quickly and Accurately Master ECG Interpretation. Philadelphia, J. B. Lippincott, 1985, p. 288, junctional rhythm.)

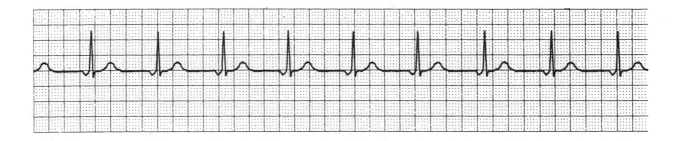

Rate_____ **Rhythm** _____

P wave_____ **PR**_____

QRS_____ **Interpretation** _____

ANSWER

Rate___71_____ **Rhythm** ___regular_____

P wave___none___ **PR**___—_____

QRS___.08_____ **Interpretation** __accelerated functional__
rhythm

Figure 4–38: Accelerated nodal rhythm (junctional tachycardia). Rhythm strip generated by the AA-700 Rhythm Simulator. (Reproduced with permission from Armstrong Medical Industries, Lincolnshire, Illinois, *DataSim*, Fig. 1.)

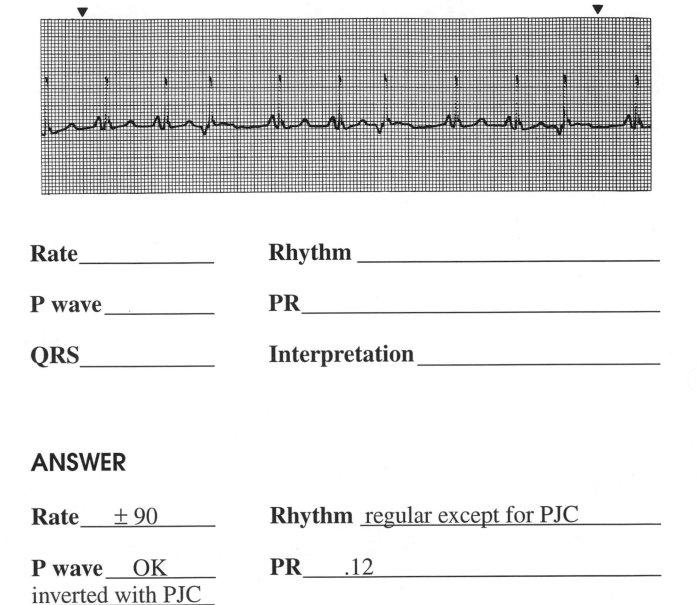

Rate_____   **Rhythm**_____

P wave_____   **PR**_____

QRS_____   **Interpretation**_____

ANSWER

Rate___±90____   **Rhythm** regular except for PJC_____

P wave___OK____   **PR**____.12_____
inverted with PJC

QRS____.06____   **Interpretation** sinus rhythm with____
                                               premature junctional complexes

Figure 4–39: Premature nodal (junctional) contraction. Note noncompensatory pause. (From Huff, J., Doernbach, D., and White, R.: ECG Workout: Exercises in Arrhythmia Interpretation, Philadelphia, J. B. Lippincott, 1985, Fig. 3.58.)

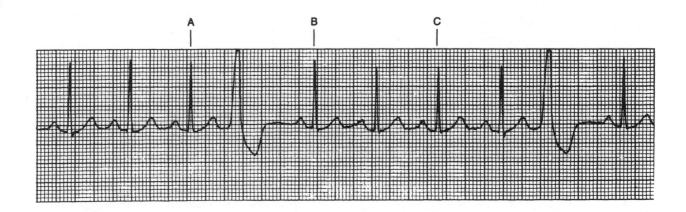

Rate_____ **Rhythm** _____

P wave_____ **PR**_____

QRS_____ **Interpretation** _____

ANSWER

Rate____±90_____ **Rhythm** regular except for PVC_____

P wave___OK_____ **PR**_____.20_____

QRS_____.06_____ **Interpretation** sinus rhythm with unifocal premature ventricular complexes

---

Figure 4–41: Unifocal premature ventricular contractions. (From Patel, J., McGowan, S., and Moody, L.: Arrythmias: Detection, Treatment, and Cardiac Drugs. Philadelphia, W. B. Saunders, 1989, Fig. 56.)

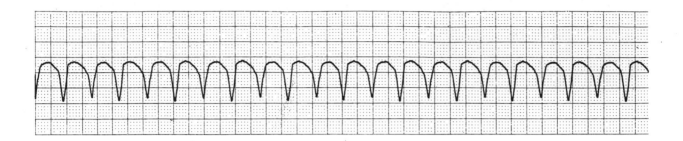

Rate_____   **Rhythm** _____

P wave_____   **PR**_____

QRS_____   **Interpretation**_____

ANSWER

Rate____167_____   **Rhythm** ___regular_____

P wave___none___   **PR**_____—_____

QRS____.12_____   **Interpretation** __ventricular tachycardia__

Figure 4–47: Ventricular tachycardia. Rhythm strip generated by the AA-700 Rhythm Simulator. (Reproduced with permission from Armstrong Medical Industries, Lincolnshire, Illinois, *DataSim*, Fig. 13.)

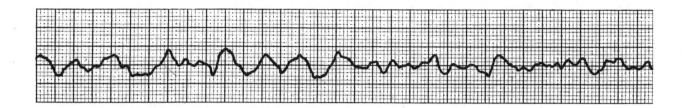

Rate_____   **Rhythm** _____

P wave_____   **PR**_____

QRS_____   **Interpretation** _____

ANSWER

Rate_____—_____   **Rhythm** ___irregular_____

P wave____—_____   **PR**____—_____

QRS_____—_____   **Interpretation** __ventricular fibrillation__

Figure 4–49: Coarse ventricular fibrillation: Rhythm strip generated by the AA-700 Rhythm Simulator. (From Patel, J., McGowan, S., and Moody, L.: Arrythmias: Detection, Treatment, and Cardiac Drugs. Philadelphia, W. B. Saunders, 1989, Fig. 84.)

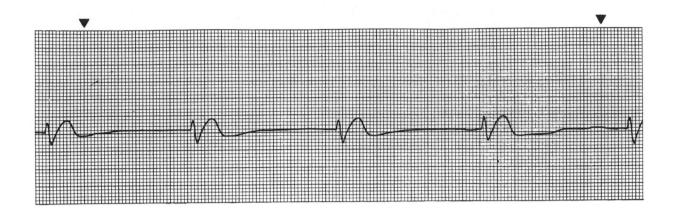

Rate_____ **Rhythm**_____

P wave_____ **PR**_____

QRS_____ **Interpretation**_____

ANSWER

Rate___36___ **Rhythm**___regular_____

P wave___—___ **PR**___—_____

QRS___.14___ **Interpretation** _idioventricular_____

Figure 4–50: Idioventricular rhythm. (From Huff, J., Doernbach, D., and White, R.: ECG Workout: Exercises in Arrhythmia Interpretation, Philadelphia, J. B. Lippincott, 1985, Fig. 4.23.)

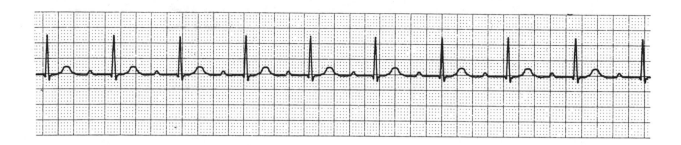

Rate_____   **Rhythm** _____

P wave_____   **PR**_____

QRS_____   **Interpretation**_____

ANSWER

Rate_____68_____   **Rhythm** ___regular_____

P wave___OK_____   **PR**____.32_____

QRS_____.06_____   **Interpretation** _sinus rhythm with____
                        first-degree AV block

Figure 4–53: First-degree block. Rhythm strip generated by the AA-700 Rhythm Simulator. (Reproduced with permission from Armstrong Medical Industries, Lincolnshire, Illinois, *DataSim*, Fig. 19.)

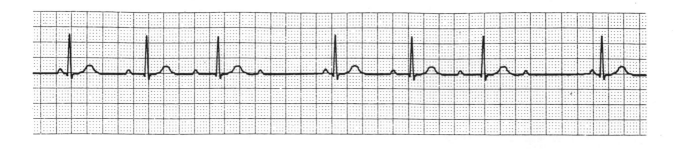

Rate_____ **Rhythm**_____

P wave_____ **PR**_____

QRS_____ **Interpretation**_____

ANSWER

Rate ± 60 **Rhythm**___irregular_____

P wave there are **PR** interval progessively lengthens_____
unconducted
P waves

QRS____.06____ **Interpretation** second-degree block
Mobitz I, Wenckebach_____

Figure 4–54: Second-degree block, Mobitz type I, or Wenckebach. Note steadily lengthening PR interval. Rhythm strip generated by the AA-700 Rhythm Simulator. (Reproduced with permission from Armstrong Medical Industries, Lincolnshire, Illinois, *DataSim*, Fig. 6.)

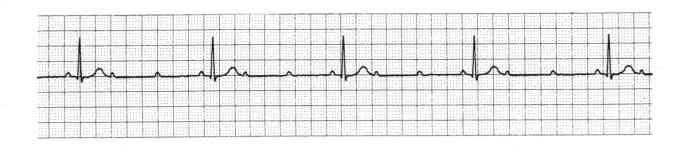

Rate_____   **Rhythm** _____

P wave_____   **PR**_____

QRS_____   **Interpretation** _____

Atrial rate _____

ANSWER

Rate_____35_____   **Rhythm** ____regular_____

P wave__unconducted P__   **PR** ____.16_____

QRS_____.08_____   **Interpretation** _second-degree___
block Mobitz II

Atrial rate__100_____

Figure 4–55: Second-degree block, Mobitz type II. Note fixed PR interval. Rhythm strip generated by the AA-700 Rhythm Simulator. (Reproduced with permission from Armstrong Medical Industries, Lincolnshire, Illinois, *DataSim*, Fig. 7.)

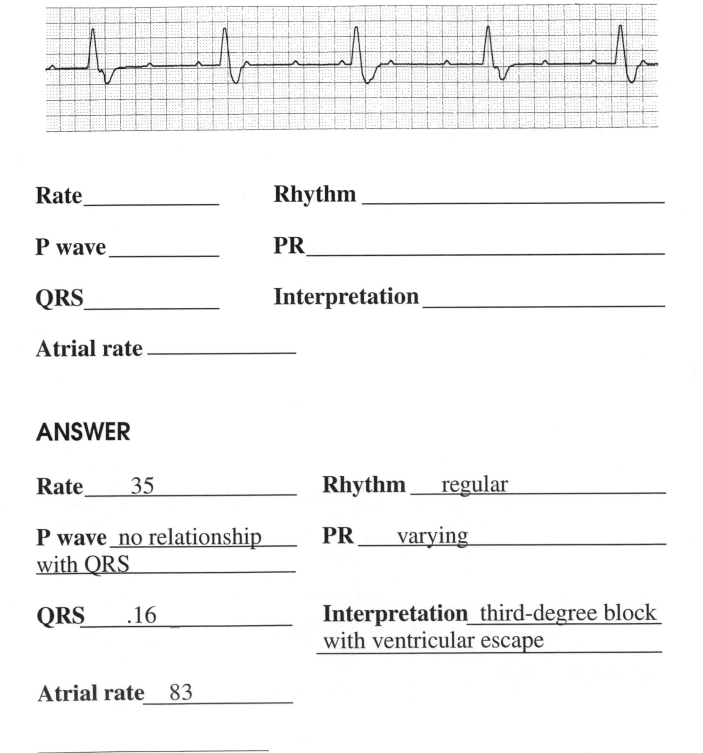

Rate_____ **Rhythm**_____

P wave_____ **PR**_____

QRS_____ **Interpretation**_____

Atrial rate_____

ANSWER

Rate_____35_____ **Rhythm**____regular_____

P wave_no relationship__ **PR**_____varying_____
with QRS

QRS_____.16_____ **Interpretation**_third-degree block_
with ventricular escape

Atrial rate___83_____

Figure 4–57: Third-degree block with ventricular excape. Rhythm strip generated by the AA-700 Rhythm Simulator. (Reproduced with permission from Armstrong Medical Industries, Lincolnshire, Illinois, *DataSim*, Fig. 8.)

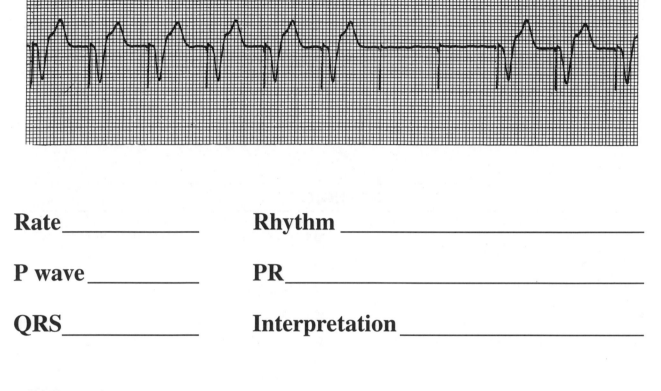

Rate_____ **Rhythm** _____

P wave_____ **PR**_____

QRS_____ **Interpretation**_____

ANSWER

Rate_____88_____ **Rhythm** regular except for period of failure to capture

P wave ___—_____ **PR** ____—_____

QRS____.16_____ **Interpretation** ventricular paced rhythm with failure to capture

Figure 4–62: Paced rhythm with failure to capture. (From Huff, J., Doernbach, D., and White, R.: ECG Workout: Exercises in Arrhythmia Interpretation, Philadelphia, J. B. Lippincott, 1985, Fig. 5.26.)

Chapter 5

Hemodynamic Monitoring

TERMINOLOGY

- Afterload
- Calibration
- Cardiac index (CI)
- Cardiac output (CO)
- Central venous pressure (CVP)
- Contractility
- Damped waveform
- Dicrotic notch
- Ejection fraction
- Embolus
- Erythrocyte
- Hemodynamics
- Intra-arterial monitoring
- Karotkoff's sounds
- Left atrial pressure (LAP)
- Leukocyte
- Mean arterial pressure (MAP)

- Mixed venous oxygen saturation (SVO_2)
- Oscilloscope
- Phlebostatic axis
- Preload
- Pulmonary artery catheter
- Pulmonary capillary wedge pressure (PCWP)
- Pulse pressure
- Thermodilution method
- Thrombosis
- Transducer
- Trendelenburg position
- Vascular resistance
- Vasoactive drugs
- Water manometer
- Zero referencing

OUTLINE

I. Hemodynamics
A. Definition

B. Basics

  1. Pressure

    a. Equation

    b. Blood pressure

      1. Systemic vascular resistance

C. Cardiac output

D. Blood and circulatory system

  1. Blood cells

  2. Blood flow

    a. Vessel diameter

    b. Cardiac control

E. Cardiac cycle

  1. Sequence blood flow

    a. Right atrium

    b. Right ventricle

    c. Pulmonary circulation

    d. Left atrium

    e. Left ventricle

      1. Stroke volume

F. Cardiac output

  1. Preload

  2. Afterload

  3. Contractility

II. Components of hemodynamic monitoring
A. Transducer

B. Amplifier

C. Display instruments

D. Catheter/tubing/flush system

E. Level

F. Balance

G. Calibration

III. Central venous pressure (CVP)
A. Definition

  1. Clinical importance

B. Measurement methods

  1. Insertion sites

  2. Water manometer

  3. Pressure transducer

C. Waveform

D. Normals

E. Resulting abnormalities

F. Complications

G. Nursing implications

    1. Accurate measurement

    2. Respiratory variation

    3. Observe complications

    4. Accurate interpretation

IV. Left atrial pressure (LAP)
    A. Definition

    1. Clinical importance

    B. Insertion

    C. Nursing implications

    1. Transducer position

    2. Respiratory cycle

    3. Positive end-expiratory pressure (PEEP)

    D. Complications

    1. Emboli

    2. Clot

    3. Infection

    E. Variables influencing

    1. Low values

    2. Elevations

    3. Trends

V. Pulmonary artery catheter
    A. Development

    B. Clinical importance

    C. Types of catheters

    1. Two lumen

    2. Three lumen

    3. Four lumen

    4. Five lumen

    5. Pacing

    6. Continuous cardiac output

    D. Nursing responsibilities

    1. Teaching

    2. Equipment

    E. Insertion method

    1. Brachial site

    2. Subclavian, internal jugular, external jugular

    3. Surgical cutdown

    4. Nursing responsibilities

    F. Clinical significance of values

    1. Pulmonary artery pressure (PAP)

      a. Systolic

      b. Diastolic

    c. Normal

  2. Pulmonary capillary wedge pressure (PCWP)

    a. Relationship to left ventricular end-diastolic pressure (LVEDP)

    b. Compared to pulmonary artery diastolic pressure (PADP)

    c. Balloon inflation

G. Complications of pulmonary artery (PA) catheters

H. Nursing implications

  1. Patient position

I. Cardiac output monitoring

  1. Equipment for intermittent thermodilution

    a. Open injectate

    b. Closed injectate

  2. Method

  3. Continuous cardiac output

  4. Clinical relevance

    a. Cardiac index (CI)

      1. Normal range

      2. Definition

      3. Low CI

        a. Causes

        b. Treatment

J. Mixed venous oxygen saturation (SVO_2)

  1. Monitoring system

2. Definition of SVO_2

3. Measurement

    a. Normal

    b. Factors affecting

      1. Decreased

      2. Increased

VI. Intra-arterial monitoring

  A. Use

  B. Equipment

  C. Waveform/measurements

    1. Systolic

    2. Diastolic

    3. Dicrotic notch

    4. Mean arterial pressure

  D. Indications for intra-arterial monitoring

  E. Complications

    1. Thrombosis

    2. Embolism

    3. Blood loss

    4. Infection

  F. Clinical considerations

    1. Difference from cuff pressure

    2. Damped waveform

  G. Nursing implications

MULTIPLE CHOICE

1. If pressure = flow × resistance, then BP = _____ × _____. Fill in the blanks.
   A. cardiac output × pulmonary vascular resistance
   B. cardiac output × systemic vascular resistance
   C. cardiac index × pulmonary vascular resistance
   D. cardiac index × systemic vascular resistance

Cardiac output (CO) = flow

Systemic vascular resistance (SVR)

Correct answer: B

Rationale: Blood pressure is affected by CO, the volume of blood that circulates through the body per minute, and SVR, the opposition to flow exerted by blood vessels.

2. Stroke volume is influenced by preload, afterload, and _____.
   A. contractility
   B. automaticity
   C. refractoriness
   D. conductivity

Correct answer: A

Rationale: Contractility is the intrinsic ability of the cardiac muscle fibers to shorten causing the ventricle to eject its stroke volume.

3. Mrs. G. has an arterial line to a transducer. In order to obtain accurate BP readings, the air-fluid interface of the stopcock must be at the phlebostatic axis, which is the level of the
   A. left atrium
   B. left ventricle
   C. right atrium
   D. right ventricle

Correct answer: C

Rationale: The phlebostatic axis is located at the fourth intercostal space, MAL.

4. An operation performed to eliminate the influence of surrounding air pressure is called
   A. zeroing
   B. leveling
   C. equating
   D. calibrating

Correct answer: A

Rationale: Zeroing is a zero reading on the monitor when the system is only sensing environmental pressure (760 mmHg at sea level).

5. A patient has a low central venous pressure (CVP). This might indicate
   A. vasoconstriction
   B. hypovolemia
   C. increased venous return
   D. increased afterload

Correct answer: B

Rationale: Hypovolemia will reduce CVP (RAP).

6. When using a transducer CVP is measured in mmHg. Measurements from a water manometer are recorded in
   A. saturation of H_2O
   B. centimeters of Hg
   C. millimeters of H_2O
   D. centimeters of H_2O

Correct answer: D

Rationale: A water manometer records centimeters of H_2O (cm H_2O), which are not equal to mmHg.

7. Your patient's CVP is elevated. To accurately interpret this data, you would
   A. call the physician
   B. reposition the transducer
   C. check lab values
   D. do a physical assessment

Correct answer: D

Rationale: CVP data are best interpreted in light of a careful physical assessment and comparison with other physiologic parameters.

8. Air or debris in the LAP catheter could cause
   A. infection
   B. cerebral embolism
   C. pneumonia
   D. pneumothorax

Correct answer: C

Rationale: Medications and fluids are not administered via the LAP catheter to decrease risk of embolic phenomena to the heart and/or brain.

9. A lower than normal LAP could be caused by
   A. excessive PEEP
   B. vasoconstriction
   C. mitral stenosis
   D. cardiac tamponade

Correct answer: A

Rationale: Hypovolemia, excessive PEEP, and massive vasodilation can lower LAP.

10. The pulmonary artery catheter allows for monitoring of
    A. right ventricle (RV) function
    B. left ventricle (LV) function
    C. left atrium (LA) function
    D. right atrium (RA) function

Correct answer: B

Rationale: LV function is indirectly monitored by the PA catheter because left ventricular end-diastolic pressure (LVEDP) is reflected in the pulmonary circulation.

11. Pulmonary artery catheter placement is verified by
    A. aspiration
    B. CT scan
    C. chest x-ray
    D. auscultation

Correct answer: C

Rationale: If fluoroscopy was not used during insertion, a chest x-ray post procedure verifies catheter placement.

12. Which pressure is directly related to LVEDP?
    A. RV
    B. pulmonary artery diastolic pressure (PADP)
    C. right atrial pressure (RAP)
    D. pulmonary artery systolic pressure (PASP)

Correct answer: B

Rationale: Pulmonary artery diastolic pressure is related to LVEDP.

13. To obtain the most reliable pressure readings, the patient's position should be
    A. contralateral
    B. lateral
    C. prone
    D supine

Correct answer: D

Rationale: Although reliable measurements may be obtained in the 90° lateral decubitus position, the reference level must be changed.

14. Cardiac index is a more precise measurement of cardiac output because it takes into account
    A. urine output
    B. lung volume
    C. body size
    D. residual volume

Correct answer: C

Rationale: $CI = L/min/m^2$, $CO = L/min$
$L/min = CO$
$m^2 = $ body surface area

15. Mr. J. has a low cardiac index. He is ordered
    A. vasopressors
    B. negative inotropes
    C. IV fluids
    D. drug aerosols

Correct answer: C

Rationale: Fluids will increase preload which will increase stroke volume.

16. Oxygen demand is determined by
    A. patient's condition
    B. arterial oxygen saturation
    C. lung function
    D. hemoglobin levels

Correct answer: A

Rationale: Oxygen demand is increased by shivering, fever, exercise, pain, and so on.

17. The dicrotic notch on the arterial waveform is caused by
    A. opening of the mitral valve
    B. closing of the mitral valve
    C. opening of the aortic valve
    D. closing of the aortic valve

Correct answer: D

Rationale: The dicrotic notch is a small notch on the downstroke of the waveform, a result of aortic valve closure.

18. To perfuse the body's vital organs, a mean arterial pressure (MAP) of _____ is required.
    A. 100 mmHg
    B. 60 mmHg
    C. 120 mmHg
    D. 80 mmHg

Correct answer: B

Rationale: Normal MAP is 70 to 100 mmHg; 60 mmHg is needed for organ perfusion.

19. The major complications of arterial pressure monitoring including thrombosis, embolism, infection, and
    A. pain
    B. scar tissue
    C. blood loss
    D. disfigurement

Correct answer: C

Rationale: Sudden dislodgment of the catheter or tubing disconnection could cause rapid blood loss.

20. Mr. B's radial artery catheter is to be discontinued. Pressure should be applied to the site for after catheter removal.
    A. 10 minutes
    B. 5 minutes
    C. 3 minutes
    D. 15 minutes

Correct answer: A

Rationale: This provides adequate hemostasis at the arterial puncture site.

CASE STUDIES

CASE STUDY #1

Ms. M. is 65 years old with a history of insulin-dependent diabetes mellitus, CVA, chronic renal insufficiency, and hypertension. She is admitted with an inferior MI.

1. Explain why Ms. M. is not a candidate for thrombolytic therapy.

   Her history of CVA and hypertension preclude the use of thrombolytics.

Ms. M. had an emergent cardiac catheter that showed 99% occlusion of the RAC, 90% occlusion of the LAD and 95% occlusion of the circumflex, and a 30% ejection fraction. An intra-aortic balloon pump (IABP) was placed via her left femoral artery and she was scheduled for CABG the next day.

2. What are the therapeutic effects of IABP therapy?

   Decreased LV work
   Increased coronary artery perfusion
   Increased LV stroke volume

After surgery, Ms. M. has a pulmonary artery catheter in place to measure her hemodynamic profile, which includes CVP, PAP, PCWP, CO, and CI.

3. What is the relationship between PAP and LV function?

   During diastole, the mitral valve is open and pressure in the left ventricle is reflected into the left atrium, as well as the pulmonary circulation.

4. Which measurement is more sensitive: CO or CI? Why?

   CO is measured in liters per minute; CI is measured in liters per minute per millimeter squared ($L/min/m^2$).
   CI is determined using the patient's height and weight (body surface area) and so is a more individualized type of measurement.

5. What effect does SVR have on CO?

   SVR = afterload
   As afterload increases, cardiac work increases. If the myocardium cannot adjust, CO will fall.

CASE STUDY #2

After three weeks at home with the flu, Miss H. arrives in the ED experiencing severe weakness. Her mucous membranes are dry, her skin turgor is poor, her BP is down, and a cardiac monitor shows sinus tachycardia. Her urine is concentrated and her lab values indicate an elevated sodium (Na) and hematocrit (Hct). A triple lumen central line is inserted due to difficulty obtaining peripheral venous access. This provides a means to measure CVP to monitor Miss H.'s fluid therapy.

1. Where is the distal tip of the catheter located to measure CVP?

    Right atrial chamber or the superior vena cava

2. What processes could cause an elevated CVP?

    Right atrial pressure elevates with a fluid overload, increased venous return or right ventricular failure such as cor pulmonale, and increased pressure in the right ventricle reflected backward as the right atrial chamber also fails.

3. As CVP changes, what changes might you assess in the patient?

    Urine volume
    Breath sounds
    Lab values: Na, Hct
    Skin changes
    Quality of pulses

4. What are the potential complications of central line insertion?

    Pneumothorax
    Infection
    Arrhythmias
    Embolic phenomenon
    Blood loss

5. Write three nursing diagnoses that describe Miss H.'s problems.

    Fluid volume deficit related to active loss (vomiting, diarrhea, poor intake).
    Potential for impaired skin integrity related to altered nutrition state.
    Activity intolerance related to generalized weakness.
    Decreased cardiac output related to alteration in preload.

Chapter 5 Case Studies

CASE STUDY #1

Ms. M. is 65 years old with a history of insulin-dependent diabetes mellitus, CVA, chronic renal insufficiency, and hypertension. She is admitted with an inferior MI.

1. Explain why Ms. M. is not a candidate for thrombolytic therapy.

Ms. M. had an emergent cardiac catheter that showed 99% occlusion of the RAC, 90% occlusion of the LAD and 95% occlusion of the circumflex, and a 30% ejection fraction. An IABP was placed via her left femoral artery and she was scheduled for CABG the next day.

2. What are the therapeutic effects of IABP therapy?

3. What is the relationship between PAP and LV function?

4. Which measurement is more sensitive: CO or CI? Why?

5. What effect does SVR have on CO?

Chapter 5 Case Studies

CASE STUDY #2

After three weeks at home with the flu, Miss H. arrives in the ED experiencing severe weakness. Her mucous membranes are dry, her skin turgor is poor, her BP is down, and a cardiac monitor shows sinus tachycardia. Her urine is concentrated and her lab values indicate an elevated sodium (Na) and hematocrit (Hct). A triple lumen central line is inserted due to difficulty obtaining peripheral venous access. This provides a means to measure CVP to monitor Miss H.'s fluid therapy.

1. Where is the distal tip of the catheter located to measure CVP?

2. What processes could cause an elevated CVP?

3. As CVP changes, what changes might you assess in the patient?

4. What are the potential complications of central line insertion?

5. Write three nursing diagnoses that describe Miss H.'s problems.

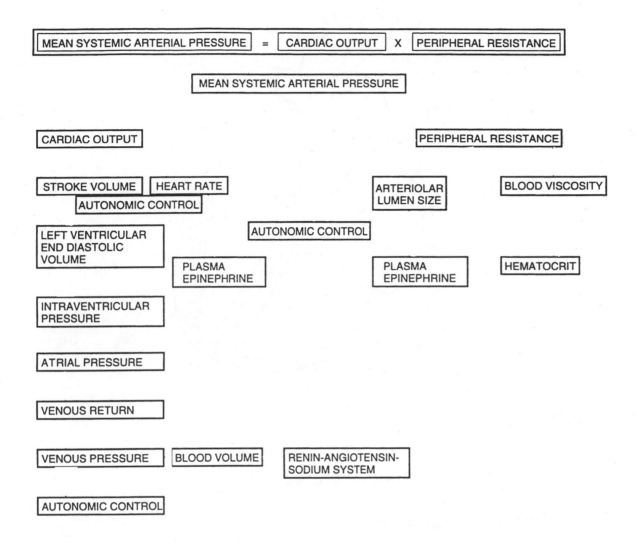

MEAN SYSTEMIC ARTERIAL PRESSURE | = | CARDIAC OUTPUT | X | PERIPHERAL RESISTANCE

MEAN SYSTEMIC ARTERIAL PRESSURE

CARDIAC OUTPUT

PERIPHERAL RESISTANCE

STROKE VOLUME   HEART RATE

AUTONOMIC CONTROL

ARTERIOLAR LUMEN SIZE

BLOOD VISCOSITY

LEFT VENTRICULAR END DIASTOLIC VOLUME

AUTONOMIC CONTROL

PLASMA EPINEPHRINE

PLASMA EPINEPHRINE

HEMATOCRIT

INTRAVENTRICULAR PRESSURE

ATRIAL PRESSURE

VENOUS RETURN

VENOUS PRESSURE   BLOOD VOLUME   RENIN-ANGIOTENSIN-SODIUM SYSTEM

AUTONOMIC CONTROL

DIRECTIONS

Place the connecting lines and arrows to show the relationship between the mechanisms that regulate systemic arterial pressure.

Figure 5–3. Mechanisms that regulate systemic arterial pressure. (From Vander, A., Sherman, J. H., and Luciano, D. S.: Human Physiology, 3rd ed. New York, McGraw-Hill, 1980. Reproduced with the permission of McGraw-Hill, Fig. 11–56, pp. 304–305.)

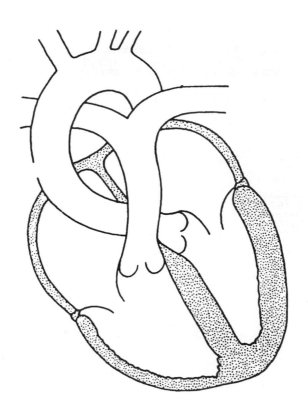

DIRECTIONS

1. Label cardiac chambers and vessels

2. Include O_2 saturation—%

   pressure—mmHg

3. Indicate where you would measure

   PAP with a ★

   CVP with an ✗

Figure 5–14. Schematic illustration of heart model depicting the pressure and oxygen saturation measurements in the various chambers of the heart. (From Gardner, P. E., and Woods, S. L.: Hemodynamic monitoring. *In:* Underhill, S. L., et al.: *Cardiac Nursing*, 2nd ed. Philadelphia, Lippincott, 1989, Fig. 34–1, p. 452.)

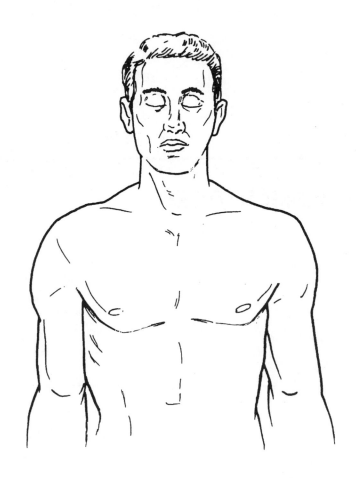

DIRECTIONS

1. Mark correct hand placement for external compressions

2. Mark anterior paddle placement sites

Figure 7–10. Paddle placement for defibrillation. (Redrawn from Sheehy, S. B.: Mosby's Manual of Emergency Care. St. Louis, C. V. Mosby, 1990, Fig. 3–21, p. 76.)

Chapter 6

Ventilatory Assistance

TERMINOLOGY

- Arterial blood gases (ABGs)
- Assist/control ventilation (A/C)
- Barotrauma
- Bicarbonate ion (HCO_3^-)
- Biot's respirations
- Bradypnea
- Buffer system
- Cheyne-Stokes respiration
- Compliance
- Continuous positive airway pressure (CPAP)
- Controlled mechanical ventilation (CMV)
- Crackles
- Diffusion
- End-tidal carbon dioxide (etCO$_2$)
- Endotracheal tube (ETT)
- Hyperinflation
- Hyperoxygenation
- Hyperventilation

- Intermittent mandatory ventilation (IMV)
- Kussmaul's respirations
- Manual resuscitation bag (MRB)
- Mechanical ventilation
- Metabolic alkalosis
- Metabolic acidosis
- Nasopharyngeal airway
- Oral airway
- Oxygen saturation (SaO$_2$)
- Oxyhemoglobin dissociation curve
- Partial pressure of arterial carbon dioxide (PaCO$_2$)
- Partial pressure of oxygen (PaO$_2$)
- Peak inspiratory pressure (PIP)
- Perfusion
- pH
- Pleural friction rub
- Pneumothorax
- Positive pressure ventilation
- Positive end-expiratory pressure (PEEP)

- Pressure support ventilation (PSV)
- Pressure-cycled ventilator
- Pulse oximetry (SpO_2)
- Respiratory alkalosis
- Respiratory acidosis
- Sigh
- Subcutaneous emphysema
- Tachypnea
- Tidal volume

- Time-cycled ventilator
- Tracheostomy tube
- Ventilation
- Ventilator settings
- Vital capacity
- Volume-cycled ventilator
- Weaning
- Wheezes

OUTLINE

I. Anatomy
  A. Primary function

  B. Upper airway

  C. Lower airway

    1. Airway

    2. Cilia

    3. Alveoli

  D. Lungs

II. Physiology
  A. Pressure changes

  B. Gas exchange

    1. Ventilation

    2. Diffusion of pulmonary capillaries

    3. Perfusion

    4. Diffusion of cells

  C. Regulation of breathing

  D. Work of breathing

    1. Compliance

    2. Static compliance

    3. Dynamic compliance

    4. Resistance

  E. Lung volumes

    1. Tidal volume

    2. Inspiratory reserve volume (IRV)

    3. Expiratory reserve volume (ERV)

    4. Residual volume (RV)

  F. Lung capacities

    1. Inspiratory capacity (IC)

    2. Functional residual capacity (FRC)

3. Vital capacity

4. Total lung capacity

III. Assessment
A. Health history

B. Physical exam

1. Inspection

a. Accessory muscles

b. Cyanosis

c. Breathing pattern

1. Eupnea

2. Tachypnea

3. Bradypnea

4. Cheyne-Stokes respiration

5. Kussmaul's respiration

6. Biot's respiration

7. Apneustic

2. Palpation

a. Subcutaneous crepitus

b. Tactile fremitus

3. Percussion

a. Resonance

b. Dullness

c. Flatness

d. Hyperresonance

e. Tympany

4. Auscultation

a. Stethoscope

1. Diaphragm

2. Bell

b. Procedure

c. Breath sounds

1. Vesicular

2. Bronchial

3. Bronchovesicular

4. Decreased

5. Adventitious

a. Crackles

b. Wheezes

c. Pleural friction rub

d. Voice sounds

1. Bronchophony

2. Egophony

3. Whispered pectoriloquy

C. Arterial blood gas interpretation

1. How obtained

2. Oxygenation

   a. Partial pressure of arterial oxygen (PaO_2)

      1. Definition

      2. Normal range

   b. Arterial oxygen saturation of hemoglobin (SaO_2)

      1. Definition

      2. Normal range

   c. Hypoxemia

   d. Relationship of PaO_2 and SaO_2

   e. Oxyhemoglobin dissociation curve

      1. Shift to right

      2. Shift to left

3. Ventilation/acid-base status

   a. pH

      1. Definition

      2. Normal range

      3. Alkalemia

      4. Acidemia

   b. Partial pressure of arterial carbon dioxide ($PaCO_2$)

      1. Definition

      2. Normal range

      3. Above normal

      4. Below normal

   c. Bicarbonate ion (HCO_3)

      1. Definition

      2. Normal range

      3. Above normal

      4. Below normal

4. Buffer system

   a. Blood

   b. Respiratory

   c. Renal

5. Interpretation

   a. Evaluate O_2

      1. PaO_2

      2. SaO_2

   b. Evaluate acid-base status

      1. pH

      2. $PaCO_2$

      3. HCO_3

   c. Determine primary acid-base imbalance

   d. Determine compensation

D. Noninvasive assessment of gas exchange

  1. Assessment of oxygenation

    a. Pulse oximetry

    b. Transcutaneous PO_2

  2. Assessment of ventilation

    a. Transcutaneous CO_2

    b. End tidal CO_2

IV. Oxygen administration
  A. Commonly used devices

    1. Nasal cannula

    2. Face mask

    3. Face masks with reservoirs

      a. Partial rebreather

      b. Nonrebreather

    4. Venturi mask

    5. Bag-valve device (BVD)

V. Airway management
  A. Positioning

  B. Oral airways

  C. Nasopharyngeal airways

  D. Endotracheal intubation

    1. Types

    2. Indications

  3. Procedures for oral intubation

    a. Sniffing position

    b. Size of endotracheal tube

    c. Laryngoscope

    d. Time of procedure

    e. Placement

  E. Nasotracheal intubation

  F. Complications

  G. Tracheostomy

    1. Indications

    2. Types

      a. Cuffed

      b. Fenestrated

      c. Cuffless

  H. Endotracheal suctioning

    1. Indications

    2. Frequency

    3. Techniques

VI. Mechanical ventilation
  A. Indications

  B. Types

    1. Noninvasive methods

a. Negative pressure

b. Noninvasive positive pressure

2. Positive pressure

a. Time-cycled

b. Pressure-cycled

c. Volume-cycled

C. Modes of mechanical ventilation

1. Controlled ventilation

a. Definition

b. Indications

2. Assist/control (A/C) ventilation

a. Definition

b. Indications

c. Complications

3. Intermittent mandatory ventilation (IMV) and synchronized intermittent mandatory ventilation (SIMV)

a. Definition

b. Indications

D. Adjuncts to mechanical ventilation

1. Positive end-expiratory pressure (PEEP)

a. Definition

b. Indications

c. Range

2. Continuous positive airway pressure (CPAP)

a. Definition

b. Delivery

c. Indications

3. Pressure support ventilation

a. Definition

b. Indications

E. Advanced methods and modes of mechanical ventilation

F. Ventilator settings

1. Tidal wave

2. Respiratory rate

3. Fraction of inspired oxygen (FiO_2)

4. Sigh

5. Sensitivity

6. Inspiratory : expiratory ratio

7. Peak inspiratory pressure (PIP)

8. Pressure limits

G. Respiratory monitoring during mechanical ventilation

1. Spontaneous tidal volume

2. Vital capacity

3. Negative inspiratory force

4. Compliance

   a. Estimated

   b. Measured

   c. Static

   d. Dynamic

   e. Changed by

H. Complications of mechanical ventilation

  1. Pulmonary

   a. Barotrauma

    1. Definition

    2. Occurrence

    3. Types

   b. Right mainstem intubation

   c. Endotracheal tube (ETT) out of position/ unplanned extubation

   d. Tracheal damage

   e. Problems with O_2 administration

   f. Acid-base disturbances

   g. Aspiration

   h. Infection

   i. Ventilator dependence/inability to wean

2. Cardiovascular

3. Gastrointestinal

4. Endocrine

5. Psychosocial

I. Nursing care

J. Medications

  1. Analgesics

   a. Indications

   b. Agents

  2. Sedatives

   a. Indications

   b. Agents

  3. Neuromuscular blocking agents

   a. Indications

   b. Agents

K. Troubleshooting

  1. Important rules

  2. Volume alarms

  3. Pressure alarms

L. Weaning from mechanical ventilation

  1. Assessment for readiness

  2. Team approach

3. Methods

  a. IMV/SIMV

  b. T piece

  c. Pressure support

  d. CPAP

4. Procedure

5. Discontinuance of weaning

6. Causes of impaired weaning

7. Terminal weaning

MULTIPLE CHOICE

1. Ventilation is defined as the movement of gases in and out of the
   A. trachea
   B. bronchioles
   C. alveoli
   D. pleural space

Correct answer: C

Rationale: Ventilation is the movement of O_2 and CO_2 in and out of the alveoli.

2. Normally, respirations are stimulated by
   A. increased CO_2 levels
   B. decreased O_2 levels
   C. decreased CO_2 levels
   D. increased O_2 levels

Correct answer: A

Rationale: High CO_2 levels stimulate the respiratory center, carotid arteries, and aorta to send messages to the medulla to regulate respiration.

3. Compliance increases with
   A. obesity
   B. pulmonary fibrosis
   C. ARDS
   D. emphysema

Correct answer: D

Rationale: The enlarged air spaces that occur with emphysema cause increased compliance.

4. The amount of air remaining in the lungs after maximum expiration is
   A. expiratory reserve volume
   B. residual volume
   C. inspiratory reserve volume
   D. tidal volume

Correct answer: B

Rationale: The average RV is 1200 ml.

5. Deep, regular respirations usually more than 20 per minute are
   A. Cheyne-Stokes
   B. apneustic
   C. Biot's
   D. Kussmaul's

Correct answer: D

Rationale: Kussmaul's respirations commonly occur with conditions that cause metabolic acidosis.

6. Percussion of emphysematous lungs produces
   A. dullness
   B. resonance
   C. hyperresonance
   D. tympany

Correct answer: C

Rationale: Hyperresonance produces a slight musical sound heard over tissue that has an increased amount of air.

7. The presence of crackles usually indicates
   A. air passing through narrow airways
   B. inflammation of the pleura
   C. lung consolidation
   D. fluid in the alveoli and airways

Correct answer: D

Rationale: Crackles are short, explosive, nonmusical, discontinuous sounds.

8. The SaO_2 refers to the relationship of O_2 to
   A. lung function
   B. metabolism
   C. hemoglobin
   D. respiratory rate

Correct answer: C

Rationale: SaO_2 refers to the amount of oxygen bound to hemoglobin.

9. A shift to the right of the oxyhemoglobin dissociation curve occurs with
   A. acidemia
   B. alkalemia
   C. CO poisoning
   D. septic shock

Correct answer: A

Rationale: A shift to the right results in more O_2 supplied to the tissues due to decreased hemoglobin affinity for O_2.

10. A $PaCO_2$ greater than 45 mmHg indicates
    A. metabolic acidosis
    B. metabolic alkalosis
    C. respiratory acidosis
    D. respiratory alkalosis

Correct answer: C

Rationale: $PaCO_2$ greater than 45 mmHg indicates CO_2 retention.

11. The blood buffer system is activated as
    A. H^+ changes
    B. HCO_3^- changes
    C. O_2 changes
    D. CO_2 changes

Correct answer: A

Rationale: As H^+ increases pH falls, resulting in acidosis and causing HCO_3^- to combine with H^+.

12. Interpret the following ABGs:

    pH 7.2, $PaCO_2$ 25, PaO_2 95, HCO_3 18
    A. respiratory acidosis
    B. metabolic acidosis
    C. respiratory acidosis with partial compensation
    D. metabolic acidosis with partial compensation

Correct answer: D

Rationale: The pH is abnormal and compensatory mechanisms are noted: $PaCO_2$ less than 35.

13. End tidal CO_2 assesses
    A. respiration
    B. ventilation
    C. oxygenation
    D. resuscitation

Correct answer: B

Rationale: Ventilation is assessed by CO_2 measurements.

14. An open airway is best maintained by
    A. nasopharyngeal airway
    B. oropharyngeal airway
    C. bag-valve device
    D. head tilt/chin lift

Correct answer: D

Rationale: The first method for maintaining a patient's airway is proper head position, using the AHA recommended head tilt/chin lift.

15. A laryngoscope is used to
    A. open the airway
    B. maintain head tilt
    C. visualize the vocal cells
    D. visualize the trachea

Correct answer: C

Rationale: A laryngoscope enables the practitioner to visualize the larynx for intubation.

16. Endotracheal suctioning
    A. depresses the cough reflex
    B. should be performed every two hours
    C. stimulates mucus production
    D. decreases intracranial pressure

Correct answer: C

Rationale: Suctioning stimulates the cough reflex and increases mucus production.

17. To facilitate tracheal suctioning you would
    A. increase airway pressure
    B. keep the patient dehydrated
    C. instill 3 to 5 cc normal saline
    D. use aerosolized mucolytics

Correct answer: D

Rationale: Studies do not support saline instillation; instead keep the patient hydrated and use aerosolized mucolytics.

18. The most commonly used positive pressure ventilators are
    A. time-cycled
    B. pressure-cycled
    C. volume-cycled
    D. inspiration-cycled

Correct answer: C

Rationale: Volume-cycled ventilators provide inspiratory flow until a preset volume has been reached.

19. If Mr. S. develops tachypnea on a ventilator that is set in the assist/control mode, he will become
    A. tired
    B. acidotic
    C. paralyzed
    D. alkalotic

Correct answer: D

Rationale: If a patient's respiratory rate is too high, he or she may develop respiratory alkalosis.

20. An indication that the ventilated patient has decreased lung compliance would be
    A. decreased PIP
    B. increased PIP
    C. increased TV
    D. decreased FiO_2

Correct answer: B

Rationale: Increasing peak inspiratory pressures indicate decreasing lung compliance or increasing lung resistance.

21. Neuromuscular blocking agents cause
    A. paralysis
    B. sedation
    C. analgesia
    D. decreased anxiety

Correct answer: A

Rationale: Neuromuscular blocking agents only provide paralysis. Patients will still require pain medications, sedation, and so on.

22. Adequate respiratory muscle strength for weaning is indicated by
    A. respiratory rate under 25/min
    B. negative inspiratory force over -10 cm H_2O
    C. spontaneous tidal volume of 2 ml/kg
    D. vital capacity of 4–5 ml/kg.

Correct answer: B

Rationale: To indicate readiness for weaning, the readings should be: negative inspiratory force -20 cm H_2O, spontaneous tidal volume 4–5 ml/kg and vital capacity 10–15 ml/kg.

CASE STUDIES

CASE STUDY #1

Mr. J., 55 years old, arrests when he has an MI. He is a smoker with early bronchitis. He is intubated and placed on a volume-cycled ventilator set at AC 16, TV 750, FiO_2 1.0.

1. Describe the difference between volume-cycled and pressure-cycled ventilators.

   Volume cycled: inspiratory phase over when preset TV (CC) is reached.

   Pressure cycled: inspiratory phase over when preset pressure (cm H_2O) is reached.

2. How is TV determined?

   Patient's weight and disease process

ABGs are drawn in 30 minutes. The results are pH 7.53, pCO_2 3.0, pO_2 210, HCO_3 24, and O_2 sat 100%.

3. Interpret these ABGs. What ventilator changes might be made and why?

   Respiratory alkalosis: pO_2 is high. Mr. J. is breathing too fast, so decrease the respiratory rate and FiO_2.

The ventilator settings are changed to AC 12, TV 750, FiO_2 .60. ABGs are drawn in one hour. The results are pH 7.48, pCO_2 30, pO_2 150, HCO_3 25, and O_2 sat 99%.

4. Interpret these ABG levels. What system is most affected by acid-base imbalances?

   Respiratory alkalosis/Central nervous system:

   - Alkalosis leads to CNS overexcitability.

   - Acidosis leads to CNS depression.

Mr. J. is awake now in sinus tachycardia with PVCs. He moves all extremities, pupils are equal and react to light, and he has spontaneous respirations at 20/minute. Ventilator settings are changed to SIMV 8, TV 750, FiO_2 .40.

5. What is the difference between A/C and SIMV and how does SIMV assist in the weaning process?

   A/C provides ventilator assistance with every breath Mr. J. initiates and has backup control if he is apneic or his respiratory rate falls below a preset rate.

   SIMV allows him to breathe on his own between ventilator breaths.

   SIMV rates can be gradually decreased allowing the patient to breathe increasingly on his or her own.

6. Provide a possible sequence for Mr. J.'s weaning process.

   IMV 4

   IMV 0

   T-tube, 40%

   Aerosol face mask, 40%

CASE STUDY #2

Mr. T. has been a COPD patient for many years. He is admitted with exacerbation of COPD and pneumonia. He is in acute respiratory distress. Current ABGs are pH 7.167, pCO_2 85, pO_2 50, HCO_3 40, O_2 sat 68%, BE/D +5.5.

1. What are the signs of respiratory distress?

   Nasal flaring

   Use of accessory muscles

   Intercostal retraction

   Abdominal breathing

   Decreased pulmonary air flow

2. Interpret Mr. T.'s ABGs. Why is his HCO_3 elevated?

   Respiratory acidosis with hypoxemia: HCO_3 is elevated due to renal compensation.

Because he is quickly losing consciousness and his breathing is so labored, Mr. T. is intubated immediately.

3. Name two ways to ascertain correct ETT placement.

   Listen for bilateral equal breath sounds

   Chest x-ray—ETT should be 2 cm above carina.

Mr. T. is suctioned for copious amounts of thick secretions and drug therapy is initiated including antibiotics and steroids.

4. How do you expect the ventilator to improve Mr. T.'s ABGs?

   Improve oxygenation with positive pressure breaths to increase pO_2.

   Improve ventilation by decreasing pCO_2.

One hour after he is intubated, Mr. T. begins to wake up and "fight" the ventilator. He is placed on a neuromuscular blocking agent to enable the provision of optimum therapy.

5. Use of neuromuscular blockade requires ventilator-assisted breathing. What other provisions are necessary?

   Sedation

   Pain control

   Opportunity to communicate

   Meticulous skin care and positioning

Chapter 6 Case Studies

CASE STUDY #1

Mr. J., 55 years old, arrests when he has an MI. He is a smoker with early bronchitis. He is intubated and placed on a volume-cycled ventilator set at AC 16, TV 750, FiO_2 1.0.

1. Describe the difference between volume-cycled and pressure-cycled ventilators.

2. How is TV determined?

ABGs are drawn in 30 minutes. The results are pH 7.53, pCO_2 3.0, pO_2 210, HCO_3 24, and O_2 sat 100%.

3. Interpret these ABGs. What ventilator changes might be made and why?

ABGs are drawn in one hour. The results are pH 7.48, pCO_2 30, pO_2 150, HCO_3 25, and O_2 sat 99%.

4. Interpret these ABG levels. What system is most affected by acid-base imbalances?

Mr. J. is awake now in sinus tachycardia with PVCs. He moves all extremities, pupils are equal and react to light, and he has spontaneous respirations at 20/minute. Ventilator settings are changed to SIMV 8, TV 750, FiO_2 .40.

5. What is the difference between A/C and SIMV and how does SIMV assist in the weaning process?

6. Provide a possible sequence for Mr. J.'s weaning process.

Chapter 6 Case Studies

CASE STUDY #2

Mr. T. has been a COPD patient for many years. He is admitted with exacerbation of COPD and pneumonia. He is in acute respiratory distress. Current ABGs are pH 7.167, pCO_2 85, pO_2 50, HCO_3 40, O_2 sat 68%, BE/D +5.5.

1. What are the signs of respiratory distress?

2. Interpret Mr. T.'s ABGs. Why is his HCO_3 elevated?

Because he is quickly losing consciousness and his breathing is so labored, Mr. T. is intubated immediately.

3. Name two ways to ascertain correct ETT placement.

Mr. T. is suctioned for copious amounts of thick secretions and drug therapy is initiated including antibiotics and steroids.

4. How do you expect the ventilator to improve Mr. T.'s ABGs?

One hour after he is intubated, Mr. T. begins to wake up and "fight" the ventilator. He is placed on a neuromuscular blocking agent to enable the provision of optimum therapy.

5. Use of neuromuscular blockade requires ventilator-assisted breathing. What other provisions are necessary?

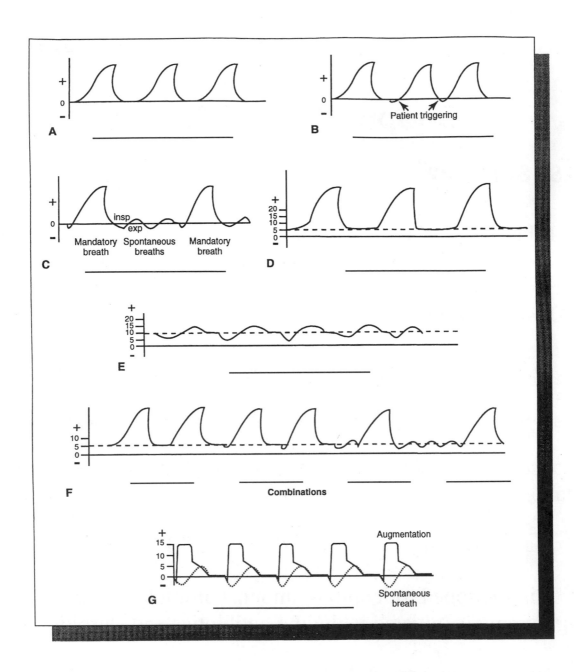

A

B Patient triggering

C insp exp
Mandatory breath   Spontaneous breaths   Mandatory breath

D

E

F Combinations

G Augmentation
Spontaneous breath

DIRECTIONS

Describe these ventilator breathing patterns.

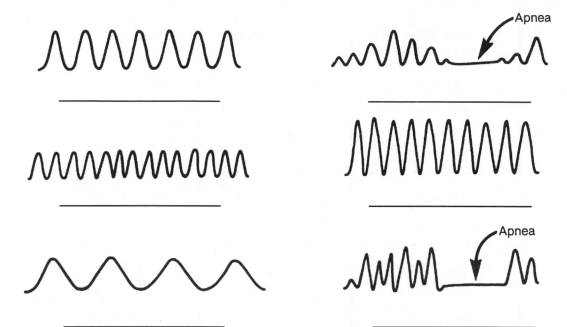

_____

_____

_____

_____

_____

_____

DIRECTIONS

Label the breathing patterns.

When might each breathing pattern be seen?

Figure 6–8. Breathing patterns. (Adapted from Kersten, L. D.: Comprehensive Respiratory Nursing, Philadelphia, W. B. Saunders, 1989, Fig. 12–28, p. 279.)

	PaCO2 < 35	PaCO2 35–45	PaCO2 > 45
HCO$_3$ < 22	pH > 7.45 _____ pH < 7.35 _____	pH < 7.35 _____	pH < 7.35 _____ or _____
HCO$_3$ 22–26	pH > 7.45 _____	pH 7.35–7.45 normal	pH < 7.35 _____
HCO$_3$ > 26	pH > 7.45 _____ or _____	pH > 7.45 _____	pH < 7.35 _____ pH > 7.45 _____

DIRECTIONS

Fill in the blanks with the correct acid-base imbalance.

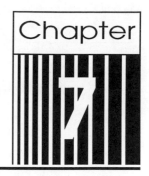

Chapter 7

Code Management

TERMINOLOGY

- Advanced cardiac life support (ACLS)
- ACLS algorithm
- Automatic implantable cardioverter defibrillator (AICD)
- Automatic external defibrillator (AED)
- Basic life support (BLS)
- Cardioversion
- Code/arrest
- Crash cart

- Defibrillation
- External pacer (TCP)
- Joules/watt-seconds
- Paradoxical pulse
- Patient Self Determination Act (PSDA)
- Pericardial tamponade
- Pericardiocentesis
- Tension pneumothorax

OUTLINE

I. Code
    A. Description

    B. Role of American Heart Association

        1. BLS

        2. ACLS

    C. Role of caregivers

1. Code team

    a. Director

    b. Nurses

        1. Primary

        2. Secondary

3. Supervisor

c. Anesthesiologist/nurse anesthetist

d. Respiratory therapist

e. Pharmacist/pharmacy technician

f. ECG technician

g. Chaplain

h. Other personnel

D. Crash cart

1. Equipment

a. Backboard

b. Monitor/defibrillator

c. Bag-valve device

d. Airway supplies

e. Drugs

II. Resuscitation efforts
A. Basic cardiac life support (BCLS)

1. Purpose

2. ABCs

a. Airway

1. Assessment

2. Head tilt/chin lift

b. Breathing

1. Assessment

2. Mouth-to-mouth

3. Alternative techniques

4. Rate

c. Circulation

1. Assessment

2. Compressions

a. Hand placement

b. Rate

c. Ventilation/compression ratio

B. Advanced cardiac life support (ACLS)

1. Primary survey

2. Secondary survey

3. Airway

4. Breathing

5. Circulation

6. Differential diagnosis

C. Recognition and treatment of dysrhythmias

1. Ventricular fibrillation (VF) and pulseless ventricular tachycardia (VT)

a. Critical actions

1. Initiate A, B, C, Ds

2. Defibrillation sequence

3. Intubate

4. Epinephrine

5. Defibrillate

6. Medications

7. Reassess

2. Pulseless electrical activity (PEA)

  a. Determine probable cause

  b. Critical actions

    1. Initiate ABCD

    2. Consider cause

    3. Epinephrine

    4. Secondary survey

3. Asystole

  a. Critical actions

    1. CPR, intubate, IV access

    2. Confirmation

    3. Ventilation

    4. Consider cause

    5. Transcutaneous pacing (TCP)

    6. Medications

    7. Termination

4. Symptomatic bradycardia

  a. Types

  b. Critical actions

    1. Assess ABC

    2. Atropine

    3. Identify rhythm

    4. TCP

    5. BP support

    6. Lidocaine

5. Symptomatic tachycardias

  a. Critical actions

    1. ABCD survey

    2. Recognize unstable tachycardia

    3. Premedicate

    4. Synchronized cardioversion

D. Electrical therapy

  1. Defibrillation

    a. Use

    b. Definition

    c. Procedure

      1. Energy

      2. Safety

    d. Complications

  2. Cardioversion

    a. Definition

    b. Difference from defibrillation

    c. Procedure

  3. Automated external defibrillator (AED)

    a. Definition

    b. Procedure

  4. Special situations

    a. Defibrillation of patient with implantable cardioverter/defibrillator

    b. Defibrillation of patient with permanent pacemaker

  5. Transcutaneous cardiac pacing

    a. Definition

    b. Procedure

E. Code drugs

  1. Determination of drugs

  2. Goals

  3. Procedure

  4. Oxygen

    a. Indications

    b. Delivery

  5. Epinephrine

    a. Action

    b. Indications

    c. Dosage

    d. Administration

  6. Atropine

    a. Action

    b. Indications

    c. Dosage

  7. Lidocaine

    a. Action

    b. Indications

    c. Dosage

    d. Administration

    e. Adverse effects

  8. Procainamide

    a. Action

    b. Indications

    c. Dosage

    d. Administration

    e. Adverse effects

  9. Bretylium tosylate

a. Action

b. Indications

c. Dosage

d. Administration

e. Adverse effects

10. Adenosine

   a. Action

   b. Indications

   c. Dosage

   d. Adverse effects

11. Verapamil

   a. Action

   b. Indications

   c. Dosage

   d. Adverse effects

12. Diltiazem

   a. Action

   b. Indications

   c. Dosage

13. Magnesium

   a. Action

   b. Indications

c. Dosage

d. Administration

e. Adverse effects

14. Sodium bicarbonate

   a. Action

   b. Indications

   c. Dosage

15. Dopamine

   a. Action

     1. 1–2 mcg/kg/min

     2. 2–10 mcg/kg/min

     3. More than 10 mcg/kg/min

     4. More than 20 mcg/kg/min

   b. Indications

   c. Dosage

   d. Adverse effects

16. Calcium chloride

   a. Action

   b. Indications

   c. Dosage

   d. Adverse effects

17. Morphine

a. Action

b. Indications

c. Dosage

III. Special problems during a code
A. Tension pneumothorax

1. Description

2. Signs and symptoms

3. Diagnosis

4. Treatment

B. Pericardial tamponade

1. Description

2. Signs and symptoms

3. Diagnosis

4. Treatment

IV. Documentation of code events
V. Care of patient after resuscitation
A. Monitoring

B. Drugs

C. Cerebral resuscitation

1. Definition

2. Goals

3. Ventilatory support

4. Other measures

D. Emotional support

VI. Psychosocial, legal, and ethical concerns
A. Psychosocial concerns

1. Family

2. Roommate

3. Staff

B. Legal and ethical concerns

1. Living will

2. Do not resuscitate (DNR) order

3. Communication

MULTIPLE CHOICE

1. A back board is placed under the patient who arrests to
   A. prevent cervical spinal injury
   B. provide a firm flat surface for chest compressions
   C. provide a means to move the patient
   D. prevent accidental shock when defibrillated

Correct answer: B

Rationale: CPR cannot be properly performed on a mattress; a hard level surface is needed for external chest compressions.

2. Without adequate oxygen, brain damage occurs within
   A. 1–2 minutes
   B. 2–3 minutes
   C. 4–6 minutes
   D. 8–10 minutes

Correct answer: C

Rationale: Brain damage occurs within 4–6 minutes; brain death occurs in 10 minutes.

3. To assess for breathlessness, the rescuer should
   A. shake and shout
   B. palpate the carotid
   C. auscultate the chest
   D. look, listen, and feel

Correct answer: D

Rationale: Look at the chest for movement, listen for air movement, and feel for exhaled air.

4. An adult who is not breathing but has a pulse should be ventilated
   A. once every 6 seconds
   B. 16 times per minute
   C. once every 3 seconds
   D. 12 times per minute

Correct answer: D

Rationale: Rescue breathing is performed 12 times per minute or once every 5 seconds.

5. In advanced cardiac life support, the primary survey includes steps A-B-C-D. "D" refers to
   A. early defibrillation
   B. disrobe the victim
   C. do not resuscitate
   D. defer to EMS personnel

Correct answer: A

Rationale: "D" refers to early defibrillation that can be accomplished with an automated external defibrillator (AED) or a conventional defibrillator.

6. An intubated patient is ventilated
   A. after every fifth compression
   B. during the fifth compression
   C. asynchronously 12–15 times per minute
   D. asynchronously 20–22 times per minute

Correct answer: C

Rationale: Ventilation of the intubated patient should not be synchronized to chest compression but performed asynchronously 12–15 times per minute.

7. Mr. T. is found unresponsive and pulseless in his driveway. The first thing you should do is
   A. give two rescue breaths
   B. call EMS
   C. shake and shout
   D. begin compressions

Correct answer: B

Rationale: As soon as unresponsiveness is determined, EMS should be called to make a defibrillator and drugs available.

8. Asystole is a rhythm that requires
   A. defibrillation
   B. atropine
   C. CPR
   D. lidocaine

Correct answer: C

Rationale: Asystole requires confirmation in more than one monitoring lead, CPR, intubation, and IV access.

9. Mr. S. is bradycardic with frequent PVCs. He is symptomatic and first requires
   A. lidocaine
   B. epinephrine
   C. atropine
   D. pacemaker

Correct answer: C

Rationale: Atropine 0.5 to 1 mg IV is the initial drug of choice.

10. Your newly admitted patient with blunt chest trauma becomes unresponsive and pulseless. You expect his rhythm to be
    A. pulseless electrical activity (PEA)
    B. ventricular tachycardia (VT)
    C. asystole
    D. sinus bradycardia (SB)

Correct answer: A

Rationale: PEA may be caused by cardiac tamponade, which could be the result of blunt chest trauma.

11. Paddle placement for anterior defibrillation is
    A. 2 ICS, RSB and 4 ICS, LMCL
    B. 4 ICS, RSB and 5 ICS, LMCL
    C. 2 ICS, LSB and 5 ICS, LMCL
    D. 2 ICS, RSB and 5 ICS, LMCL

Correct answer: D

Rationale: Paddle position for anterior or transverse defibrillation is 2 ICS, RSB and 5 ICS LMCL.

12. Electrical energy for defibrillation is measured in
    A. milliamperes
    B. joules
    C. watt-minutes
    D. alternating current

Correct answer: B

Rationale: The amount of energy delivered is measured in joules or watt-seconds.

13. Symptomatic tachyarrhythmias are treated with cardioversion. These symptoms include
    A. flushed skin, headache, increased urine output
    B. decreased urine output, decreased BP
    C. decreased level of consciousness, decreased BP, cool clammy skin
    D. rapid pulse, increased BP

Correct answer: C

Rationale: These are symptoms related to low cardiac output caused by the tachyarrhythmia.

14. The release of the charge in cardioversion is synchronized with
    A. T wave
    B. R wave
    C. P wave
    D. U wave

Correct answer: B

Rationale: A defibrillator set in the synchronous mode for cardioversion senses the R waves to deliver the charge in the QRS.

15. Your patient is to receive an implanted cardioverter-defibrillator (ICD). He wonders if it will be safe to sleep with his wife. You know that
    A. He should be very careful not to touch anyone when it discharges.
    B. He should not defibrillate.
    C. His wife may feel the shock.
    D. His wife may become unresponsive.

Correct answer: C

Rationale: There is no danger to people if the ICD discharges while the patient is touching them, although the shock, which is comparable to the sensation of contact with an electric outlet, may be felt by the other person.

16. Epinephrine increases myocardial oxygen demand by
    A. increasing afterload
    B. decreasing heart rate
    C. increasing preload
    D. decreasing contractility

Correct answer: A

Rationale: Epinephrine is a potent vasoconstrictor, increasing systemic vascular resistance and arterial blood pressure.

17. The antiarrhythmic drug of choice for ventricular ectopy is
    A. Pronestyl
    B. Bretylium
    C. Quinidine
    D. Lidocaine

Correct answer: D

Rationale: Lidocaine is first line for PVC, VT, and VF.

18. Mrs. S. has just begun treatment with Verapamil to slow her heart rate. You know she is a borderline congestive heart failure (CHF) patient, so you assess her for
    A. bounding pulses
    B. hypotension
    C. hypertension
    D. rapid respirations

Correct answer: B

Rationale: Verapamil causes vasodilation and decreased cardiac contractility along with a decreased heart rate.

19. A patient who suffers an arrest becomes acidotic for two reasons. These are:
    A. retention of CO_2 and accumulation of nitrogenous wastes
    B. hyperoxygenation and accumulation of organic acids
    C. retention of CO_2 and accumulation of organic acids
    D. hyperoxygenation and accumulation of nitrogenous wastes

Correct answer: C

Rationale: CO_2 is retained due to inadequate ventilation; organic acids accumulate due to anaerobic metabolism induced by hypoxia.

20. Dopamine is to be infused at 5 mcg/kg/min. The patient weighs 175 lbs. The concentration is dopamine 400 mg in 250 cc D_5W. How many cc/hr will be given?
    A. 14.9 cc/hr
    B. 100 cc/hr
    C. 15.5 cc/hr
    D. 56.2 cc/hr

Correct answer: A

Rationale:
$$\frac{cc}{hr} = \frac{250\ cc}{400\ mg} \times \frac{1\ mg}{1000\ mg} \times \frac{5\ mg}{1\ kg} \times \frac{1}{min} \times$$
$$\frac{1\ kg}{2.2\ lb.} \times \frac{175\ lb.}{1} \times / \frac{60\ min}{1\ hour} = 14.91\ \frac{cc}{hr}$$

CASE STUDIES

CASE STUDY #1

You are running up the steps, late for work, when you find a man collapsed in the stairway. As you pull him to the closest landing, you are rapidly remembering the steps of basic life support (i.e., CPR). You remember to shake and shout to assess for unresponsiveness. Since he did not arouse, you go to the nearest phone and call EMS.

1. Why is it so important to call EMS even before beginning CPR?

    EMS brings defibrillation equipment and drugs. Rapid defibrillation, according to the American Heart Association, is the link in the chain of survival that is most likely to improve survival rates.

2. How long does an adult who is not breathing have before brain damage begins?

    Brain damage begins in four minutes; after six minutes brain damage will almost always occur; after ten minutes brain death is certain.

Upon your return, you begin the ABCs of CPR.

A = airway   You do a head tilt/chin lift to pull his tongue off the back of his throat.

B = breathing

3. Describe the process of artificial ventilation.

    Look, listen, and feel to determine breathlessness.

    If victim is not breathing:
    - Pinch the nostrils closed
    - Maintain head tilt/chin lift
    - Make a tight seal around victim's mouth with your mouth
    - Give two slow breaths; watch for victims chest to rise
    - Allow victim to exhale between breaths

C = circulation

4. Describe the technique for external cardiac compressions.

    Determine pulselessness by feeling carotid

    If there is no pulse:
    - Position heel of hand on lower third of the sternum
    - Compress the chest straight downward
    - Depress sternum 1 ½ to 2 inches, 80 to 100 times per minute
    - Cycle 15 compressions then 2 breaths

5. The EMS crew arrives and they are unable to obtain IV access. Which drugs can be given via the endotracheal tube? Why is this route effective?

A - atropine

L - lidocaine

E - epinephrine

Drugs are absorbed via alveolar capillary blood supply. Dosage via this route is 2 to 2.5 times the normal dose.

6. A member of the crew looks in the victim's wallet for identification and finds a living will that states "No CPR." What should be done?

The American Heart Association states in its guidelines for discontinuing basic life support that life support should be discontinued if "a valid no-CPR order is presented to the rescuers."

(*Textbook of Basic Life Support for Healthcare Providers*, 1994, American Heart Association.)

CASE STUDY #2

Mr. B. collapses on the golf course. He is unresponsive, not breathing, and pulseless. CPR is initiated. The EMS crew arrives and puts Mr. B. on the monitor. He is in ventricular fibrillation and is defibrillated twice before his rhythm changes to atrial fibrillation. His pulses are now palpable and he is awake.

Later in the CCU, Mr. B.'s heart rate jumps to 135, he complains of shortness of breath and lightheadedness, and his monitor shows SVT. After vagal maneuvers and drugs are unsuccessful, the decision is made to try cardioversion.

1. Describe the hemodynamic effects of ventricular fibrillation.

Numerous pieces of ventricular tissue depolarizing and repolarizing at their own rates make the ventricle quiver instead of contracting in a coordinated manner, resulting in no cardiac output.

2. The steps in the algorithm to treat ventricular fibrillation require defibrillation three times with increasing joules. What is the purpose of defibrillation?

Defibrillation depolarizes the entire myocardium at one time, wiping out any electrical activity. Hopefully, the sinus node will repolarize first and take over as the pacemaker.

3. Describe the differences between defibrillation and cardioversion using chart format.

	Defibrillation	Cardioversion
Urgency	Emergency	Elective
Performed by	Anyone trained: RN, EMT, MD	Physician
Rhythm	Ventricular fibrillation, pulseless ventricular tachycardia	Symptomatic tachyarrhythmias
Starting joules	200, then 300, then 360	50 to 100
Charge release	When buttons are pushed	Synchronized to discharge within QRS complex

4. Before Mr. B. is cardioverted, he is given a short-acting hypnotic. When the charge is released, he moans and "jumps." Does he feel the shock? What is happening?

Cardioversion causes myocardial depolarization just like defibrillation but affects not only myocardial cells but all of the muscles including the diaphragm. Therefore, as the diaphragm contracts after depolarization, Mr. B. moans; and, as his skeletal muscles contract after depolarization, he "jumps."

5. Because cardioversion is usually elective, what do you tell Mr. B. prior to the procedure? Do not use the word "shock."

Show Mr. B. a rhythm strip, explaining the process of sending an electrical message to his heart to slow it down. Speak in terms of his symptomatology: how he feels now and how he will feel later.

Chapter 7 Case Studies

CASE STUDY #1

You are running up the steps, late for work, when you find a man collapsed in the stairway. As you pull him to the closest landing, you are rapidly remembering the steps of basic life support (i.e., CPR). You remember to shake and shout to assess for unresponsiveness. Since he did not arouse, you go to the nearest phone and call EMS.

1. Why is it so important to call EMS even before beginning CPR?

2. How long does an adult who is not breathing have before brain damage begins?

Upon your return, you begin the ABCs of CPR.

      A = airway   You do a head tilt/chin lift to pull his tongue off the back of his throat.

      B = breathing

3. Describe the process of artificial ventilation.

      C = circulation

4. Describe the technique for external cardiac compressions.

5. The EMS crew arrives and they are unable to obtain IV access. Which drugs can be given via the endotracheal tube? Why is this route effective?

6. A member of the crew looks in the victim's wallet for identification and finds a living will that states "No CPR." What should be done?

Chapter 7 Case Studies

CASE STUDY #2

Mr. B. collapses on the golf course. He is unresponsive, not breathing, and pulseless. CPR is initiated. The EMS crew arrives and puts Mr. B. on the monitor. He is in ventricular fibrillation and is defibrillated twice before his rhythm changes to atrial fibrillation. His pulses are now palpable and he is awake.

Later in the CCU, Mr. B.'s heart rate jumps to 135, he complains of shortness of breath and lightheadedness, and his monitor shows SVT. After vagal maneuvers and drugs are unsuccessful, the decision is made to try cardioversion.

1. Describe the hemodynamic effects of ventricular fibrillation.

2. The steps in the algorithm to treat ventricular fibrillation require defibrillation three times with increasing joules. What is the purpose of defibrillation?

3. Describe the differences between defibrillation and cardioversion using chart format.

4. Before Mr. B. is cardioverted, he is given a short-acting hypnotic. When the charge is released, he moans and "jumps." Does he feel the shock? What is happening?

5. Because cardioversion is usually elective, what do you tell Mr. B. prior to the procedure? Do not use the words "electric" or "shock."

Chapter 8

Shock

TERMINOLOGY

- Acute tubular necrosis (ATN)
- Anaerobic metabolism
- Anaphylactic shock
- Capillary refill
- Cardiogenic shock
- Catecholamines
- Chronotropism
- Colloid
- Crystalloid
- Cyanosis
- Disseminated intravascular coagulation (DIC)
- Distributive shock
- Fluid challenge
- Hemodilution
- Hydrostatic pressure
- Hypovolemic shock
- Intra-aortic balloon pump (IABP)

- Leukopenia
- Microcirculation
- Military antishock trousers (MAST)
- Multiple organ failure (MOF)
- Neurogenic shock
- Osmotic pressure
- Peritoneal lavage
- Plasma expander
- Positive inotrope
- Prodromal
- Septic shock
- Shock
- Systemic vascular resistance (SVR)
- Third spacing
- Thrombolytic
- Vagolytic drug
- Vasopressor

OUTLINE

I. Introduction
   A. Definition

   B. Overall effects

II. Anatomy and physiology review
   A. Cardiovascular system

      1. Vessels

      2. Function

   B. Microcirculation

      1. Description

      2. Function

   C. Blood flow

      1. Resistance

   D. Essential circulatory components

III. Classifications of shock
   A. Hypovolemic

      1. Definition

      2. Causes

         a. Hemorrhage

         b. External fluid loss

         c. Internal volume deficits

      3. Results

   B. Cardiogenic

      1. Definition

      2. Causes

      3. Pathophysiology

   C. Obstructive

      1. Definition

      2. Hemodynamics

   D. Distributive

      1. Definition

      2. Neurogenic

         a. Definition

         b. Causes

      3. Anaphylactic

         a. Definition

         b. Pathophysiology

      4. Septic

         a. Definition

         b. Causes

         c. Pathophysiology

         d. Toxic shock syndrome

      5. Relative hypovolemia

IV. Stages of shock
  A. Initial

    1. Description

    2. Reversal

  B. Early or compensatory

    1. Description

    2. Neural compensation

    3. Endocrine compensation

    4. Chemical compensation

  C. Intermediate or progressive

    1. Description

    2. Systemic circulation

    3. Microcirculation

  D. Refractory or irreversible

    1. Description

      a. Blood

      b. Renal

      c. Myocardial

      d. Acidosis

      e. Clotting

      f. Cerebral

    2. Cause of death

V. Assessment
  A. Importance

  B. History and prevention

    1. Description

    2. Hypovolemic shock

      a. Prevention

      b. Assessment

    3. Cardiogenic

      a. Prevention

      b. Therapies

    4. Obstructive

      a. Prevention

      b. Therapies

    5. Distributive

      a. Prevention

        1. Neurogenic

        2. Anaphylactic

        3. Septic

      b. Assessment

VI. Clinical picture
  A. Central nervous system

  B. Cardiovascular

    1. Blood pressure

a. Cuff pressures

b. Pulses

c. Orthostatic vital signs

d. Pulsus paradoxus

2. Pulse

3. Heart sounds

4. Neck veins

5. Capillary refill

6. Central venous pressure (CVP)

7. Pulmonary artery pressure (PAP)

a. Preload

b. SVO_2

C. Respiratory

1. Description

2. Pulse oximetry

D. Renal

E. Skin and mucus membranes

F. Musculoskeletal

VII. Diagnostic tests
A. Lab studies

B. Urine

C. Chest x-rays

D. Echocardiogram

E. Diagnostic peritoneal lavage

F. Computed tomography (CT)

VIII. Nursing diagnosis
IX. Medical interventions
A. General goals

B. Hypovolemic

C. Cardiogenic

D. Obstructive

E. Distributive

F. Fluid therapy

1. IV access

2. Fluid challenge

3. Types fluids

a. Crystalloids

b. Colloids

1. Albumin/plasmanate

2. Dextran

3. Hespan

c. Blood and blood products

1. Access and procedure

2. Goal

3. Whole blood

4. Packed red cells

5. Fresh frozen plasma

6. Platelets

X. Pharmacologic therapy
   A. Drugs that affect contractility

   1. Positive inotropes

   2. Negative inotropes

   B. Drugs that affect preload

   C. Drugs that affect afterload

   D. Drugs that alter rate

   E. Oxygen

   F. Antibiotics

   G. Steroids

   H. Sodium bicarbonate

XI. Mechanical management
   A. Intra-aortic balloon pump (IABP)

   B. Ventricular assist device (VAD)

C Pneumatic antishock garment (PASG)

XII. Nursing interventions
   A. Airway

   B. Positioning

   C. Maintaining body temperature

   D. Maintaining skin integrity

   E. Psychological support

   F. Patient outcomes

XIII. Complications
   A. Central nervous system (CNS)

   B. Cardiovascular

   C. Respiratory

   D. Renal

   E. Hepatic

   F. Gastrointestinal

   G. Multiple organ dysfunction syndrome (MODS)

MULTIPLE CHOICE

1. The portion of the vascular bed most significant for cell survival is
   A. pulmonary circulation
   B arteriole
   C. microcirculation
   D. systemic circulation

Correct answer: C

Rationale: Microcirculatory functions include delivering nutrients to the cells, removing waste from the cells, and regulating blood volume.

2. Blood flow is facilitated by
   A. vessel diameter
   B. blood viscosity
   C. vessel length
   D. changing pressures

Correct answer: D

Rationale: Flow is opposed by resistance, which is determined by vessel length, blood viscosity, and vessel diameter.

3. Shock is a life-threatening response to alterations in
   A. circulation
   B. respiration
   C. elimination
   D. mentation

Correct answer: A

Rationale: Alterations in circulation result in impaired tissue oxygenation and cellular metabolism.

4. The majority of cases of cardiogenic shock are caused by
   A. pancreatitis
   B. anaphylaxis
   C. acute myocardial infarction (AMI)
   D. gastrointestinal (GI) bleed

Correct answer: C

Rationale: Cardiogenic shock occurs when diseased coronary arteries are not capable of meeting the O_2 demand of working myocardial cells.

5. Obstructive shock occurs when there is a mechanical obstruction to _____ blood flow.
   A. portal
   B. peripheral
   C. pulmonary
   D. central

Correct answer: D

Rationale: Obstructive shock occurs when the heart or great vessels are compressed.

6. When neurogenic shock occurs, interruption in sympathetic nerve impulses causes
   A. hypertension
   B. vasodilation
   C. hyperventilation
   D. bradycardia

Correct answer: B

Rationale: Disturbance in sympathetic nerve impulses causes vasodilation which decreases SVR, venous return, preload, and CO.

7. Vasodilation occurring in distributive shock results in
   A. decreased heart rate
   B. increased venous return
   C. decreased preload
   D. increased afterload

Correct answer: C

Rationale: See question 6.

8. The substances released from cellular breakdown mediated by the antigen-antibody reaction cause
   A. hypovolemia
   B. increased capillary permeability
   C. vasoconstriction
   D. relaxation of smooth muscle

Correct answer: B

Rationale: These substances cause relative hypovolemia due to vasodilation and contraction of smooth muscle.

9. Endotoxins released by destroyed bacteria cause
   A. release of histamine
   B. decreased capillary permeability
   C. increased venous return
   D. hypertension

Correct answer: A

Rationale: Endotoxins cause the release of histamine, a vasoactive substance that causes increased capillary permeability.

10. In the initial stage of shock, decreased cardiac output results in
    A. increased sympathetic stimulation
    B. increased parasympathetic stimulation
    C. increased vagal stimulation
    D. increased urine output

Correct answer: A

Rationale: Increased sympathetic stimulation occurs in an attempt to maintain tissue perfusion.

11. In response to decreased renal perfusion, the juxtaglomerular (JG) apparatus releases
    A. angiotensin
    B. renin
    C. aldosterone
    D. antidiuretic hormone (ADH)

Correct answer: B

Rationale: Renin is released from the JG cells and reacts with angiotensin to produce angiotensin I. Renin also activates the release of ADH and aldosterone.

12. The classic signs and symptoms of shock appear in which stage?
    A. initial
    B. early
    C. intermediate
    D. refractory

Correct answer: C

Rationale: Activation of compensatory mechanisms in the early stages of shock mask the classic signs and symptoms.

13. Blood pooling in the capillary bed and arterial blood pressure too low to support perfusion of vital organs causes
    A. CNS disturbances
    B. pancreatitis
    C. pneumonia
    D. multiple organ failure (MOF)

Correct answer: D

Rationale: Prolonged inadequate tissue perfusion contributes to MOF.

14. The first system to be affected by changes in cellular perfusion is
    A. cardiovascular
    B. central nervous
    C. respiratory
    D. gastrointestinal

Correct answer: B

Rationale: The CNS is the most sensitive to changes in the supply of O_2 and nutrients.

15. If the brachial pulse is readily palpable, approximate systolic pressure is
    A. 50 mmHg
    B. 60 mmHg
    C. 70 mmHg
    D. 80 mmHg

Correct answer: D

Rationale: A palpable femoral pulse means the systolic pressure is approximately 70 mmHg and a palpable carotid means the SBP is 60 mmHg.

16. The most sensitive method of assessing oxygenation in shock is
    A. pulse oximetry
    B. ABG
    C. auscultation
    D. capillary refill

Correct answer: B

Rationale: Because peripheral circulation is decreased, ABG may be required.

17. The primary treatment for distributive shock is
    A. relieve obstruction
    B. restore circulating volume
    C. restore vascular tone
    D. reestablish myocardial circulation

Correct answer: C

Rationale: Interventions are directed toward reversing the relative hypovolemia caused by vasodilation.

18. A fluid challenge typically involves the rapid infusion of _____ to change BP or CVP.
    A. 100 cc normal saline (NS)
    B. 100 cc plasma
    C. 250 cc NS
    D. 250 cc plasma

Correct answer: C

Rationale: The initial infusion is usually 250 to 500 cc NS.

19. Large volume crystalloid infusion could be accomplished with which of the following
    A. plasmanate
    B. dextran
    C. albumin
    D. lactated Ringer's

Correct answer: D

Rationale: Lactated Ringer's closely resembles plasma.

20. Fresh frozen plasma (FFP) is administered to replace
    A. clotting factors
    B. platelets
    C. white cells
    D. red cells

Correct answer: A

Rationale: FFP replaces all clotting factors except platelets.

CASE STUDIES

CASE STUDY #1

Mr. R., 53 years old with a history of peptic ulcer disease, develops a massive GI bleed. By the time he arrives in the emergency department, he is cool, pale, diaphoretic, and tachycardic, with weak, thready pulses. His BP falls and he becomes increasingly lethargic. Fluid resuscitation is begun immediately via two large-bore antecubital IV catheters.

1. Shock is a state of inadequate circulation that causes faulty cellular metabolism. What is necessary for adequate circulation?

    fluid volume—intravascular

    cardiac pump

    vessels with tone

Mr. R.'s GI bleed is under control but his hemodynamic status is deteriorating. This is characteristic of the progressive stage of shock in which intrinsic factors are thought to be the cause of the worsening condition.

2. How does inadequate circulation interfere with cellular metabolism?

    Decreased circulation causes decreased O_2 and nutrients to cells, which causes aerobic metabolism to change to anaerobic metabolism which greatly decreases production of adenosine triphosphate and increases formation of metabolic acids.

3. Mr. R.'s hemoglobin and hematocrit (H&H) is used to determine his fluid therapy. What is the relationship between H&H and fluid choice?

    Hematocrit determines whether the patient needs fluid or cells:

      - Optimal O_2 carrying capacity is HCT 35–45

      - HCT < 20: patient needs cells (i.e., blood)

      - HCT > 55: patient needs fluid (i.e., plasma, NS)

4. Mr. R.'s hematocrit is now 58 after multiple units of RBCs. Does he require crystalloids or colloids? Describe the difference.

    Crystalloids are electrolyte solutions that move freely out of vascular space; for example, if you infuse two liters, only 500 cc remains in vascular space.

    Colloids are fluids containing molecules large enough to be retained in blood vessels.

    Without aggressive therapy, shock moves rapidly to the irreversible stage, in which therapies are ineffective. This is largely due to microcirculatory failure and failure of the adjacent cells.

5. Describe microcirculation and its function.

    Microcirculation is the end point of the circulatory transport system between arteriole and venule. It is the largest organic unit in the body, comprising 90% of all blood vessels. Microcirculation operates on demand and at any one time contains only 6–7% total blood volume. No feedback mechanism exists between systemic circulation and microcirculation, so as shock progresses, systemic circulation constricts, microcirculation dilates, and pooling occurs.

CASE STUDY #2

Ms. L. becomes short of breath and her heart rate, blood pressure, respiratory rate, and temperature increase. She is warm and pink and noticeably apprehensive. Blood cultures are positive for gram-negative cocci. The physician explains to her husband that she is in septic shock.

1. Later, her husband comes to you and asks how can she be in shock if she is pink and warm because he thought people in shock are cold, clammy, and pale. What is your explanation?

   In words Mr. L. can understand, explain the pathophysiology of massive vasodilation caused by bacterial toxins acting directly on the vessels causing them to lose their tone.

Antibiotics are begun, as are fluids and vasopressors, as Ms. L.'s BP begins to fall.

2. What caused the initial increased BP and the eventual decrease in BP?

   Initial sympathetic compensatory response maintains the BP at or higher than normal. Eventually compensatory vasoconstriction can no longer maintain status quo.

3. What are possible complications of vasopressor therapy?

   Complications include constriction, which could shut down nutrient flow to the tissues and organs.

Invasive access and monitoring lines are placed. Ms. L. is intubated and placed on a mechanical ventilator.

4. Shock is a total body response. What is the relationship between shock and the GI system?

   The GI system plays a role in the irreversibility of shock. The poorly perfused liver cannot detoxify as it should. The poorly perfused bowel becomes ischemic and the intestinal wall breaks down allowing bacteria to move to the rest of the body (translocation).

5. As time passes and Ms. L.'s condition worsens, her husband tells you that she never wanted to live like this. He asks you what an advance directive is.

   Advanced directives provide for decision making once a person is incompetent to make his or her own decisions and is terminally ill. It can be a living will and/or a surrogate decision maker, and is specifically defined by law in each state.

Chapter 8 Case Studies

CASE STUDY #1

Mr. R., 53 years old with a history of peptic ulcer disease, develops a massive GI bleed. By the time he arrives in the emergency department, he is cool, pale, diaphoretic, and tachycardic, with weak, thready pulses. His BP falls and he becomes increasingly lethargic. Fluid resuscitation is begun immediately via two large-bore antecubital IV catheters.

1.   Shock is a state of inadequate circulation that causes faulty cellular metabolism. What is necessary for adequate circulation?

Mr. R.'s GI bleed is under control but his hemodynamic status is deteriorating. This is characteristic of the progressive stage of shock in which intrinsic factors are thought to be the cause of the worsening condition.

2.   How does inadequate circulation interfere with cellular metabolism?

3.   Mr. R.'s hemoglobin and hematocrit (H&H) is used to determine his fluid therapy. What is the relationship between H&H and fluid choice?

4.   Mr. R.'s hematocrit is now 58 after multiple units of RBCs. Does he require crystalloids or colloids? Describe the difference.

5.   Describe microcirculation and its function.

Chapter 8 Case Studies

CASE STUDY #2

Ms. L. becomes short of breath and her heart rate, blood pressure, respiratory rate, and temperature increase. She is warm and pink and noticeably apprehensive. Blood cultures are positive for gram-negative cocci. The physician explains to her husband that she is in septic shock.

1. Later, her husband comes to you and asks how can she be in shock if she is pink and warm because he thought people in shock are cold, clammy, and pale. What is your explanation?

Antibiotics were begun as were fluids and vasopressors as her BP began to fall.

2. What caused the initial increased BP and the eventual decrease in BP?

3. What are possible complications of vasopressor therapy?

Invasive access and monitoring lines are placed. Ms. L. is intubated and placed on a mechanical ventilator.

4. Shock is a total body response. What is the relationship between shock and the GI system?

5. As time passes and Ms. L.'s condition worsens, her husband tells you that she never wanted to live like this. He asks you what an advance directive is.

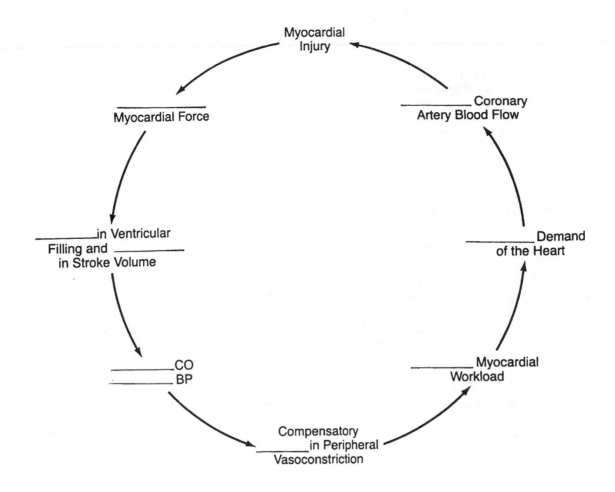

Figure 8–2. Cycle of cardiogenic shock.

DIRECTIONS

Fill in the blanks with either increased, ↑, or decreased, ↓.

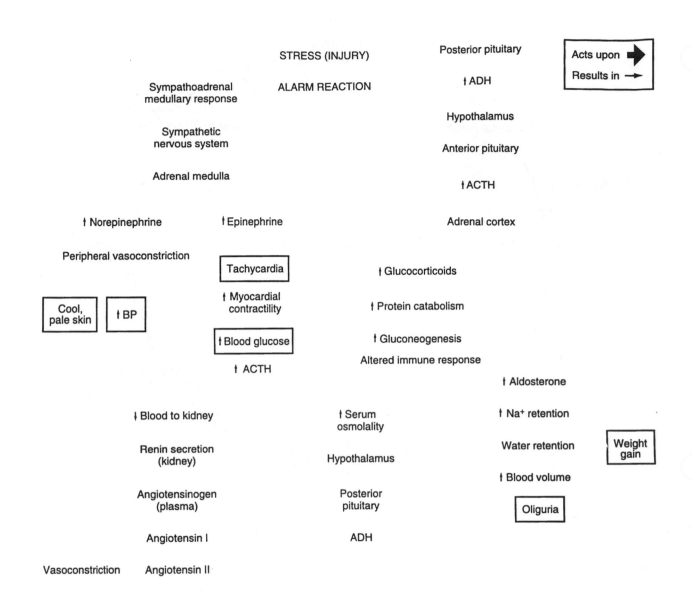

DIRECTIONS

Make the connections using the arrow key at the top of the flow-chart.

Figure 8–4. Physiologic response to stressors in shock. (From Polaski, A. L., and Tatro, S. E.: Luckmann's Core Principles and Practice of Medical-Surgical Nursing, Fig. 56–3.)

Parameter	Cardiogenic	Hypovolemic	Obstructive	Distributive
				Septic Anaphylactic Neurogenic
Cardiac Output (CO) NR 4–8 L/min				
Cardiac Index (CI) NR 2.8–4.2 L/min/m^2				
Right atrial pressure (RAP) NR 0–8 mmHg				
Pulmonary artery diastolic pressure (PADP) NR 4–12 mmHg				
Pulmonary capillary wedge pressure (PCWP) NR 1–10 mmHg				
Systemic vascular resistance (SVR) NR 900–1400 dyne/sec/cm^{-5}				
Mixed venous oxygen saturation (SVO$_2$) NR 60–80%				

Abbreviations: NR—normal range

DIRECTIONS

Fill in hemodynamic alterations (i.e., high, low) in each column.

Cardiac Alterations

TERMINOLOGY

- Angina
- Antidysrhythmics
- Atheroma
- Automaticity
- Autotransfusion
- Baroreceptors
- Cardiac reserve
- Chemoreceptors
- Conductivity
- Congestive heart failure (CHF)
- Coronary artery bypass graft (CABG)
- Coronary artery disease (CAD)
- Endocardium
- Epicardium
- Excitability
- Hyperlipidemia
- Infective endocarditis
- Insufficiency

- Murmur
- Myocardial infarction (MI)
- Myocardium
- Nitrates
- Palpitations
- Percutaneous transluminal coronary angioplasty (PTCA)
- Pulmonary edema
- Rhythmicity
- S_1
- S_2
- S_3
- S_4
- Stroke volume
- Subendocardial MI
- Transmural MI
- Vasodilators

OUTLINE

I. Normal structure and function

A. Heart sounds

  1. S_1

  2. S_2

  3. S_3

  4. S_4

  5. Heart murmur

B. Autonomic control

C. Coronary circulation

D. Properties of cardiac muscle

  1. Contractility

  2. Rhythmicity

  3. Conductivity

  4. Automaticity

  5. Excitability

E. Conduction

F. Factors of circulation

  1. Cardiac output (CO) or cardiac index (CI)

  2. Stroke volume

    a. Preload

    b. Afterload

    c. Contractility

  3. Blood pressure

II. Coronary artery disease (CAD) or arteriosclerotic heart disease (ASHD)

A. Pathophysiology

B. Assessment

  1. Medical assessment

    a. Risk factors

    b. Diagnostic studies

      1. 12-lead electrocardiogram (ECG/EKG)

      2. Holter

      3. Exercise tolerance

      4. Chest x-ray

      5. Phonogram

      6. Echocardiogram

      7. Transesophageal echocardiography

      8. Radioisotope studies

      9. Cardiac catheterization/arteriography

      10. Coronary angiography

  2. Diagnostic measures

    a. Serum electrolytes

      1. Potassium

2. Calcium

3. Sodium

   b. Serum enzymes

     1. Creatine phosphokinase (CPK)

     2. Lactate dehydrogenase (LDH)

     3. Aspartate transaminase (AST)

C. Nursing diagnosis

D. Nursing interventions

E. Medical interventions

F. Outcomes

III. Angina
   A. Pathophysiology

   B. Assessment

   C. Etiology and precipitating factors

     1. CAD

     2. Coronary artery spasm

     3. Activity or stress

     4. Hypertension

     5. Anemia

     6. Dysrhythmia

     7. CHF

   D. Signs and symptoms

     1. Location pain

     2. Description

     3. Last 1–4 minutes

     4. Clenched fist

     5. Begins with exertion, ends with rest

   E. Types of angina

   F. Nursing diagnosis

   G. Medical interventions

   H. Outcomes

IV. Myocardial infarction (MI)
   A. Definition

   B. Pathophysiology

   C. Assessment

     1. Medical Assessment

       a. EKG

       b. Cardiac enzymes

   D. Diagnostic studies

     1. Coronary angiography

     2. Pyrophosphate

     3. Multigated acquisition scan (MUGA)

     4. Myocardial perfusion imaging

     5. Electrophysiological studies

E. Nursing diagnosis

F. Interventions

    1. Nursing management of complications

        a. Pericarditis

        b. Endocarditis

        c. Dressler's syndrome

    2. Medical treatment

        a. Pharmacological approach

          1. Analgesics

          2. Nitroglycerin

          3. Antiarrhythmics

            a. Type IA

            b. Type IB

            c. Type II

            d. Type III

            e. Type IV

          4. Thrombolytic therapy

          5. Streptokinase

          6. Tissue plasminogen activator (t-PA)

          7. Chewable acetylsalicylic acid (ASA)

        b. Interventional treatments

          1. Percutaneous transluminal coronary angiography

          2. Directional coronary atherectomy

          3. Intracoronary stent

          4. Excimer laser coronary angioplasty

        c. Surgical treatments

          1. Coronary artery bypass graft (CABG)

          2. Chest/mediastinal tubes

          3. Autotransfusion

          4. Intra-aortic balloon pump (IABP)

          5. Cardiac transplantation

        3. Radiofrequency catheter ablation

        4. Permanent pacemakers

        5. Implanted cardioverter-defibrillator (ICD)

        6. Outcomes

V. Congestive heart failure (CHF)

    A. Pathophysiology

        1. Left-sided

        2. Right-sided

    B. Assessment

        1. Etiology

          a. Decreased inflow blood

          b. Increased inflow blood

c. Obstructed outflow

     e. Liver function studies

d. Damaged heart muscle

    C. Nursing diagnosis

e. Increased metabolic needs

    D. Interventions

2. Precipitating factors

      1. Treatment of existing conditions

3. Diagnostic factors

      2. Preventing further or expanding complications

a. History and physical

        a. Pulmonary edema

b. Chest x-ray

        b. Cardiogenic sock

c. Hemodynamic monitoring

      3. Treating underlying causes

d. Laboratory studies

    E. Outcomes

MULTIPLE CHOICE

1. The three major coronary arteries are
   A. right interior descending, left posterior ascending, and left circumflex
   B. right interior descending, left interior descending, and right circumflex
   C. right coronary artery left interior descending and left circumflex
   D. left coronary artery left artery descending and left circumflex

Correct answer: C

Rationale: The three arteries are RCA, LID, and L circumflex.

2. The left circumflex coronary artery supplies
   A. posterior ventricular septum, part of left atrium entire posterior wall
   B. posterior ventricular septum, entire posterior wall, left atrium
   C. posterosuperior ventricular septum, part of left atrium, SA Node
   D. atrioventricular (AV) node, left atrium, posterior left ventricles

Correct answer: B

Rationale: The left circumflex supplies posterior ventricular septum, entire posterior wall left atrium.

3. In a patient with congestive heart failure, a nurse should expect to hear

    A. S_4 with bell stethoscope at the fifth intercostal

    B. S_3 with bell stethoscope at the fifth intercostal

    C. S_4 with stethoscope diaphragm at the fifth intercostal

    D. S_3 with stethoscope diaphragm at the fifth intercostal

Correct answer: A

Rationale: S_4 is heard with the bell of the stethoscope; with S_1 and S_2, it sounds like "te lubb dubb."

4. A galloping heartbeat can be heard with the bell of a stethoscope at the fifth intercostal in a patient with

    A. port MI

    B. severely failing heart

    C. fluid overload

    D. over-forceful atrial contraction

Correct answer: B

Rationale: A galloping heartbeat is heard with the bell side of the stethoscope. It is a distinguishing sound of the failing heart.

5. Optimal contractility occurs at a pulmonary capillary wedge pressure (PCWP) of

    A. 8–12 mmHg

    B. 0–8 mmHg

    C. 12–18 mmHg

    D. 18–22 mmHg

Correct answer: C

Rationale: PCWP is a measurement of left-sided preload. Refer to Starling's Law of the Heart.

6. An increase in afterload decreases CO in all of the following except

    A. vasoconstriction

    B. vasodilation

    C. semilunar valve stenosis

    D. hypertension

Correct answer: B

Rationale: Afterload refers to the resistance to blood flow during ventricular ejection. The less force the heart must overcome, the more rapidly it can contract; therefore, vasodilation increases CO.

7. The following diagnostic studies are ordered for the patient with coronary artery disease. Which identifies valvular function, measures the size of the cardiac chambers, and evaluates cardiac disease progression?

    A. 12-lead EKG

    B. echocardiogram

    C. radioisotope studies

    D. cardiac catheterization

Correct answer: B

Rationale: EKG is baseline and identifies rhythm disturbances. Echocardiogram is an *acoustic imaging* procedure. Radioisotopes show abnormal myocardial cells and cardiac catheterization measures (among other things) *pressures* within chambers.

8. Untreated hypokolemia can result in

    A. ventricular fibrillation

    B. premature ventricular contractions (PVCs)

    C. tetany

    D. irritability

Correct answer: B

Rationale: Hypokolemia results in PVCs, ventricular tachycardia, ventricular fibrillation, and death.

9. The fastest rising and falling cardiac enzyme is
    A. LDH
    B. SGOT
    C. SGPT
    D. CPK

Correct answer: D

Rationale: CPK is the fastest rising and falling enzyme—an important factor in assessing patient status.

10. Nursing interventions for the patient with CAD include teaching regarding modifiable risk factors, two of which are
    A. high-density lipoprotein (HDL) and low-density lipoprotein (LDL)
    B. age and race
    C. family history and race
    D. hyperlipidemia

Correct answer: A

Rationale: HDLP and LDLP are modifiable factors that the patient can *learn* how to change and implement with nursing assistance.

11. The physician orders antiplatelet agents to prevent problems with CAD. Identify one such agent.
    A. probucol
    B. gemfilbrozil
    C. HMG—CoA
    D. dipyridamole

Correct answer: D

Rationale: Persantine (Dipyridamole) is the only antiplatelet listed above.

12. Angina is a transient event; however, it may be a precursor to cell death from myocardial ischemia. The nurse's first action for a patient experiencing angina are
    A. assess pain, administer NTG, provide O_2
    B. provide O_2, place at rest, offer NTG
    C. administer NTG, O_2, and pain medication
    D. administer pain medication and elevate head of bed

Correct answer: A

Rationale: The nurse needs to assess, observe, and report type and degree of pain and effects of Rx on pain and VS. O_2 is given to decrease cell death.

13. Management of patients experiencing a myocardial infarction includes maintaining adequate myocardial oxygenation, decreasing myocardial workload, relieving pain and anxiety, and intervening promptly to prevent complications. One complication, that can lead to the need for valve replacement is
    A. endocarditis
    B. pericarditis
    C. Dressler's syndrome
    D. infective carditis

Correct answer: A

Rationale: Endocarditis may result in need for valve replacement. Pericarditis may result in need for pericardiectomy. Dressler's syndrome is effectively treated with ASA.

14. Patients undergoing CABG are placed on cardiopulmonary bypass during the procedure. After the graft is anastomosed, chest and mediastinal tubes are inserted. These tubes are removed when
    A. tension pneumothorax results
    B. lungs are reexpanded and negative pressure reestablished
    C. lungs are reexpanded and positive pressure reestablished
    D. pleural space is reexpanded

Correct answer: B

Rationale: Negative pressure is the normal state. Lung, not pleural space is re-expanded.

15. Distinguishing right heart failure (RHF) from left heart failure (LHF) is important in choosing the correct treatment. What signs and symptoms belong to LHF?
    A. increased heart rate and bounding pulses
    B. bounding pulses and elevated CVP
    C. murmur at apex and diaphoresis
    D. increased heart rate and oliguria

Correct answer: D

Rationale: LHF is a syndrome or symptom, not a disease. S&S—the nurse would note the following as a result of ineffective pumping action: decreased CO, blood volume remaining in LV, and accumulation of fluid in lung and pleural space, increase HR, and oliguria.

16. The IABP is used in severe CHF to
    A. decrease afterload
    B. increase preload
    C. decrease preload
    D. increase afterload

Correct answer: A

Rationale: The IABP is used to assist circulation by decreasing afterload and augmenting diastolic pressure.

17. A life-threatening form of CHF is pulmonary edema. Medications given for this include
    A. IV pentobarbital, aminophylline, and Lasix
    B. IV morphine, cysophylline, and Lasix
    C. IV morphine, aminophylline, and Bumex
    D. IV pentobarbital, cysophylline, and Bumex

Correct answer: C

Rationale: Bumex is given as a diuretic, aminophylline is given to assist in gas exchange, and IV morphine is given to increase venous capacitance.

18. An expected outcome for the patient with MI is
    A. decreased coronary artery perfusion
    B. increased coronary artery vasospasm
    C. increased coronary artery perfusion
    D. increased dysrhythmias

Correct answer: C

Rationale: The goal is coronary artery perfusion.

19. Which of the following EKG changes is indicative of ischemia?
    A. lengthened T wave
    B. elevated ST segment
    C. inverted T wave
    D. deep Q wave

Correct answer: C

Rationale: Deep Q wave reflects an *infarct*. ST elevation indicates *injury*, and T wave inversion indicates *ischemia*.

20. A concern for a patient being treated for CHF is
    A. nitrate poisoning
    B. normovolemia
    C. decreasing PCWP
    D. digitalis toxicity

Correct answer: D

Rationale: Cardiotonics (digitalis preparations) are given to CHF patients to improve CO. The nurse observes the clinical S&S of toxicity in the CHF patient (note these patients may have already been taking this Rx).

CASE STUDIES

CASE STUDY #1

Mrs. W., 85 years old, becomes pale and diaphoretic, with HR 120, R 36, BP 100/56. She has moist coarse crackles throughout her lung fields and ABGs evidence respiratory acidosis: pH 7.2, pCO_2 80, pO_2 55, O_2 sat 75%, HCO_3 30. Her chest x-ray shows pulmonary edema and an enlarged cardiac silhouette. She is intubated and placed on AC 16, TV 600, FiO_2 .60, PEEP +2.5. Morphine, digitalis, and Lasix are administered.

1. What are the compensatory mechanisms of CHF? Which are evidenced in Mrs. W.?

    Tachycardia, ventricular dilation, ventricular hypertrophy

    She is tachycardic with an enlarged cardiac silhouette.

2. What lab values should be obtained for Mrs. W. and why?

    Complete blood count (CBC) and differential to check for infection

    Hemoglobin and hematocrit to check for anemia

    Blood urea nitrogen (BUN) and creatine to check for renal failure

    Cardiac enzymes to check for MI

    Electrolytes (Na, K, CI, CO_2) to check for imbalances

3. What are the effects of digitalis on the failing heart?

    Digitalis causes sustained increase in output in the failing heart by increasing myocardial contractility.

4. Write the two primary nursing diagnoses for Mrs. W. at this time.

    Decreased cardiac output related to alteration in inotropic changes in the heart (CHF)

    Impaired gas exchange related to ventilation perfusion imbalance (CHF)

5. How would you know the medications were effective?

    Lungs clear, decreased respirations, decreased HR, increased BP, increased urine output, ABG normal, decreased pain and/or anxiety, skin warm and dry

CASE STUDY #2

Mr. J., 63-year-old white male, presents in the Emergency Department with complaints of severe chest pain that began early this morning on the way to work. He is alert and oriented, pale, and very anxious. His wife states his father and brother both died in their early 50s of heart attacks. Mr. J. is a bank executive whose corporation is in the process of reengineering. He is overweight and smokes one pack of cigarettes per day.

An initial EKG shows ST elevation in the V leads. His enzymes are within normal limits, chest x-ray clear, and heart normal. Mr. J. is admitted to CCU with a diagnosis of acute anterior MI. Tridil (nitroglycerin) is infusing at 5 mcg/minute and he is given morphine 5 mg IVP, which controls his chest pain, O_2 4L/NC, VS 134/72, 94, and 24, SR on the monitor.

The decision is made to take Mr. J. directly to the catheterization lab where a PTCA is successfully performed. A single vessel lesion in the right coronary artery was confirmed. He is returned to his room in stable condition.

1. What are the risk factors of CAD? How do they apply to Mr. J.?

   Age, sex, heredity, smoking, diet, exercise, BP, diabetes mellitus (DM)

   Mr. J. is a middle-aged, overweight smoker with a family history of CAD. Also, he is probably under a great deal of stress at work.

2. How does IV NTG control CP?

   NTG controls CP by causing venodilation, thereby decreasing venous return and myocardial O_2 demand.

3. Why is Mr. J. a candidate for PTCA?

   He has a single vessel disease and no previous MI.

4. What is the most probable reason that Mr. J.'s enzymes are within normal limits in the ED?

   It may be too early for the enzymes to be found in his blood.

5. What kind of health teaching does Mr. J. need? When should it be started?

   Mr. J.'s health teaching should be started immediately, addressing medications, diet, smoking, and exercise. He should be in a cardiac rehabilitation program.

Chapter 9 Case Studies

CASE STUDY #1

Mrs. W., 85 years old, becomes pale and diaphoretic, with HR 120, R 36, BP 100/56. She has moist coarse crackles throughout her lung fields and ABGs evidence respiratory acidosis: pH 7.2, pCO_2 80, pO_2 55, O_2 sat 75%, HCO_3 30. Her chest x-ray shows pulmonary edema and an enlarged cardiac silhouette. She is intubated and placed on AC 16, TV 600, FiO_2 .60, PEEP +2.5. Morphine, digitalis, and Lasix are administered.

1. What are the compensatory mechanisms of CHF? Which are evidenced in Mrs. W.?

2. What lab values should be obtained for Mrs. W. and why?

3. What are the effects of digitalis on a failing heart?

4. Write the two primary nursing diagnoses for Mrs. W. at this time.

5. How would you know the medications were effective?

Chapter 9 Case Studies

CASE STUDY #2

Mr. J., 63-year-old white male, presents in the Emergency Department with complaints of severe chest pain that began early this morning on the way to work. He is alert and oriented, pale, and very anxious. His wife states his father and brother both died in their early 50s of heart attacks. Mr. J. is a bank executive whose corporation is in the process of reengineering. He is overweight and smokes one pack of cigarettes per day.

An initial EKG shows ST elevation in the V leads. His enzymes are within normal limits, chest x-ray clear, and heart normal. Mr. J. is admitted to CCU with a diagnosis of acute anterior MI. Tridil (nitroglycerin) is infusing at 5 mcg/minute and he is given morphine 5 mg IVP, which controls his chest pain, O_2 4L/NC, VS 134/72, 94, and 24, SR on the monitor.

The decision is made to take Mr. J. directly to the catheterization lab where a PTCA is successfully performed. A single vessel lesion in the right coronary artery was confirmed. He is returned to his room in stable condition.

1. What are the risk factors of CAD? How do they apply to Mr. J.?

2. How does IV NTG control CP?

3. Why is Mr. J. a candidate for PTCA?

4. What is the most probable reason that Mr. J.'s enzymes are within normal limits in the ED?

5. What kind of health teaching does Mr. J. need? When should it be started?

Pathophysiology Flow Diagram
Congestive Heart Failure
Impairment of diastolic and systolic heart function

$$\downarrow CO$$

SNS
A.   Tachycardia

     ↑ Preload

B.   Vasoconstriction

     ↑ Afterload

C.   ↑ Contractility
     ↑ Myocardial oxygen demand
     ↓ Contractility

$$\downarrow BP$$

↑ Renin
↑ Angiotensin
↑ Aldosterone
↑ ADH

↑ Sodium reabsorption

↑ Blood valve

↑ Ventricular filling

Pulmonary or peripheral edema

↑ Preload

DIRECTIONS

Diagram (draw) arrows demonstrating pathophysiology.

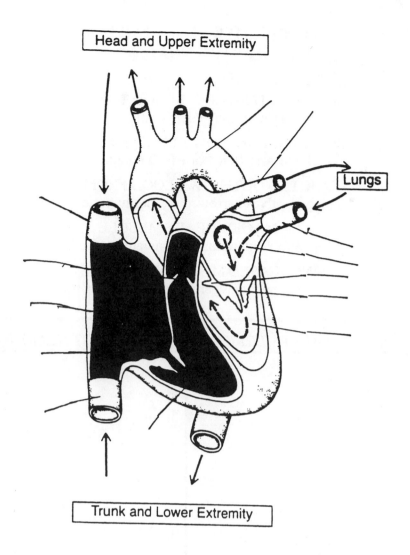

Head and Upper Extremity

Lungs

Trunk and Lower Extremity

DIRECTIONS

Label cardiac chambers and vessels.

Figure 9–4: Structure of the heart, and course of blood flow through the heart chambers. (Reproduced with permission from Guyton, A. C.: *Textbook of Medical Physiology*. 7th ed. Philadelphia, W. B. Saunders, 1986.)

CONGESTIVE HEART FAILURE
ETIOLOGY

DECREASED INFLOW BLOOD TO HEART
(Hemorrhage/dehydration)

INCREASED INFLOW BLOOD TO HEART
(Excessive fluid/Na + H_2O retention)

OBSTRUCTED OUTFLOW BLOOD FROM HEART
(Damaged valves/narrowed arteries/hypertension)

DAMAGED HEART MUSCLE
(Myocardial infarction/inflammatory process)

INCREASED METABOLIC NEEDS
(Fever/pregnancy/hypertension/chronic anemia)

Cases	LEFT HEART FAILURE	RIGHT HEART FAILURE
S&S	1. 2. 3. 4. 5. 1. 2. 3. 4. 5. 6. 7. 8. 9. 10. 11.	1. 2. 3. 1. 2. 3. 4. 5. 6. 7. 8. 9.

DIRECTIONS

Identify cardiac problems associated with left- or right heart failure. List symptoms of LHF and RHF.

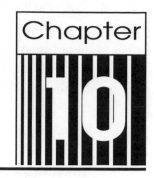

Chapter
10

Nervous System Alterations

TERMINOLOGY

- Autonomic dysreflexia
- Babinski reflex
- Cheyne-Stokes respirations
- Decerebrate
- Decorticate
- Herniation syndromes

- Increased intracranial pressure (IICP)
- Parasympathetic nervous system (PNS)
- Positive end expiratory pressure (PEEP)
- Sympathetic nervous system (SNS)
- Valsalva's maneuver

OUTLINE

---

1. Nursing assessment

   a. History

   b. Glasgow Coma Scale

   c. Neurological assessment

      1. Mental status

         a. Consciousness

         b. Language skills

         c. Memory

      2. Cranial nerve functioning

         a. Cranial nerves

         b. Spontaneous movement

         c. Muscle tone

         d. Coordination of movement

         e. Abnormal postures and reflexes

            i. Hemiplegia

            ii. Decorticate

            iii. Decerebrate

            iv. Babinski reflex

      3. Vital signs

      4. Technologies

         a. Intracranial pressure monitoring

            i. Intraparenchymal fiberoptic probe

            ii. Intraventricular catheter

            iii. Epidural probe

            iv. Subarachnoid bolt

         b. Waveform monitoring

         c. Hemodynamic monitoring

         d. Monitoring cerebral oxygenation

         e. Arterial monitoring

         f. Bedside EEG

         g. Transcranial Doppler

         h. Evoked potentials

   2. Medical assessment

C. Nursing diagnosis

D. Interventions

   1. Nursing interventions

      a. Objectives of nursing management

      b. General nursing care

         1. Antidiuretic hormone (ADH) physiology

            a. Diabetes insipidus (DI)

            b. Syndrome of inappropriate antidiuretic hormone (SIADH)

2. Medical/nonsurgical treatment

   a. Hyperventilation

   b. Diuretics

   c. Corticosteroids

   d. Oxygenation

   e. Blood pressure management

   f. Reducing metabolic demands

3. Surgical interventions

E. Nursing outcomes

II. Head injury
  A. Pathophysiology

   1. Scalp lacerations

   2. Skull fractures

    a. Linear

    b. Depressed

    c. Basilar

   3. Brain injury

    a. Primary brain injury

     1. Concussion

     2. Contusion

     3. Penetrating

     4. Diffuse axonal

    b. Secondary brain injury

     1. Hematomas

     2. Hemorrhage

     3. Herniations (see IICP)

B. Assessment

C. Nursing diagnosis

D. Interventions

   1. Nursing interventions

   2. Medical/nonsurgical

   3. Surgical

E. Outcomes

III. Spinal cord injury
  A. Pathophysiology

   1. Spinal shock

   2. Biochemical changes

   3. Vascular changes

   4. Complete versus incomplete

B. Assessment

   1. Nursing assessments

    a. Airway and respiratory status

b. Neurological assessment

c. Motor and reflex assessments

d. Sensory assessment

e. Hemodynamic assessment

f. Gastrointestinal tract assessment

g. Bowel and bladder assessment

h. Autonomic dysreflexia

i. Skin assessment

j. Psychological assessment

2. Medical assessment

C. Nursing diagnosis

D. Interventions

1. Nursing

2. Medical

E. Outcomes

IV. Acute cerebrovascular disease
    A. Pathophysiology

1. Atherosclerosis

a. Thrombus

b. Embolism

2. Hemorrhagic

a. Chronic hypertension

b. Ruptured aneurysm

c. Arteriovenous malformations

B. Assessment

1. Nursing

2. Medical

C. Nursing diagnosis

D. Interventions

1. Nursing

2. Medical/nonsurgical

3. Surgical treatment of occlusive stroke

4. Medical management of hemorrhagic cerebrovascular accident (CVA)

5. Surgical treatment of hemorrhagic CVA

E. Outcomes

V. Status epilepticus
   A. Pathophysiology

B. Assessment

1. Nursing

    2. Medical   1. Nursing

C. Nursing diagnosis   2. Medical

D. Interventions   E. Outcomes

MULTIPLE CHOICE

---

1. Intracranial compliance is a measure of
    A. cerebral edema
    B. cerebral blood flow
    C. cerebrospinal fluid (CSF) displacement
    D. the brain's compensatory mechanisms

Correct answer: D

Rationale: Intracranial compliance measures the brain's compensatory mechanisms and demonstrates the effects of volume on pressure.

2. Under normal circumstances the cerebral vasculature exhibits pressure and chemical autoregulation. What happens when autoregulation is lost?
    A. cerebral blood flow (CBF) is not affected
    B. shunting of CSF is blocked
    C. hypertension increases CBF
    D. central venous engorgement occurs

Correct answer: C

Rationale: Hypertension increases CBF and hypotension causes ischemia).

3. Herniation syndromes can be life-threatening events. Which syndrome causes the supratentorial contents to compress vital centers of the brain stem?
    A. uncal herniation
    B. central herniation
    C. tonsillar herniation
    D. cingulate herniation

Correct answer: B

Rationale: Central herniation is a downward shift of the cerebral hemispheres, basal ganglia, and diencephalon through the tentorial notch.

4. Nursing neurological assessment of the patient with increased intracranial pressure includes the Glasgow Coma Scale, history, and cranial nerve assessment. Which cranial nerves are responsible for the consensual light response, elevation of the eyelids, and eye movement?
    A. I, IX, and X
    B. III, IV, and VI
    C. II, V, and VII
    D. X, XI, and XII

Correct answer: B

Rationale: Cranial nerves III, IV, and VI work together for extraocular movements.

5. A test performed by the physician for brain stem function is the oculovestibular response (ice water calorics). The normal response to this would be
   A. the eyes move away from the ice water
   B. the eyes do not move
   C. the eyes move toward the ice water
   D. the eyes move towards the nose (midline)

Correct answer: C

Rationale: The eyes moving towards the ice water is indicative of an intact brain stem; all other responses are indicative of severe brain stem injury.

6. Abnormal posturing in response to noxious stimuli or pain indicates the location of pathology. Mr. H., a closed head injury patient, responds to painful stimuli by hyperextending his head, clenching his jaw, and extending both upper and lower extremities. This indicates a lesion in the midbrain or pons. What is this posturing called?
   A. decorticate
   B. Babinski
   C. decerebrate
   D. hemiparetic

Correct answer: C

Rationale: Decerebrate posturing or rigidity is the result of a midbrain or pons lesion.

7. Patients who experience IICP are sometimes placed on intracranial monitoring devices to assess direct measurements of ICP for better planning of care. Each device has its specific benefits and disadvantages. The intraparenchymal fiberoptic probe has which advantage and which disadvantage?
   A. therapeutic draining of CSF/risk of infection
   B. no tearing of dura mater/ inaccurate readings at high ICP
   C. ease of insertion/frequent irrigation needed to maintain patency
   D. no concern related to level of transducer/ fragility

Correct answer: D

Rationale: This type of monitor is fragile but there is no concern for the level of transducer.

8. One major complication of head injuries is diabetes insipidus (DI). Clinical symptoms of this condition include
   A. polyuria and hypernatremia
   B. dehydration and hypovolemia
   C. extreme thirst
   D. all of the above

Correct answer: A

Rationale: If the patient is alert, extreme thirst is reported; dehydration and hypovolemia are present in the patient who cannot perceive thirst. Hypernatremia is a result of hypo-osmolar state due to free water loss, and polyuria is the hallmark sign of DI.

9. Ms. P. has had a subdural hematoma removed and is one day postop. She demonstrates the following: weight gain, sodium level of 120 mEq/L, and osmolality of 235 mOsm/kg. What would you expect to see related to Ms. P.'s urinary output?

A. no change

B. low output

C. increased output

D. fluctuating

Correct answer: B

Rationale: Ms. P. is showing signs of SIADH, which causes the patient to present symptoms of water retention. Ms. P. would have low urine output.

10. Medical management of IICP includes hyperventilation either by setting the ventilator at a rate to produce hyperventilation or manual hyperventilation. Long-term use of hyperventilation is controversial. What is the purpose of hyperventilation?

A. to induce vasodilation

B. to induce vasoconstriction

C. to reduce CSF production

D. to stabilize the blood-brain barrier

Correct answer: B

Rationale: Hyperventilation is used to induce vasoconstriction; CO_2 is a potent cerebral vasodilator.

11. Patients with head injuries present different problems for family members than do other critically ill patients. One important point for the nurse to remember is that the patient's personality and cognitive changes are very devastating to the family. What is one of the most important things the nurse can do for family members?

A. limit visiting

B. provide distractions

C. provide information

D. consult a clergy member

Correct answer: C

Rationale: The nurse's role often includes providing continuity in information.

12. A common mechanism of head injuries is

A. rotation and flexion

B. acceleration and deceleration

C. hyperextension

D. flexion and extension

Correct answer: B

Rationale: This injury is a result of the moving head following a straight line and striking a stationary object.

13. One of the first responses in spinal cord injury is spinal shock. This is defined as

A. temporary loss of all functions below the level of the lesion

B. ischemia

C. incomplete lesion

D. all of the above

Correct answer: A

Rationale: Spinal shock is temporary loss of autonomic, sensory, and motor functions below the level of the lesion and is secondary to the loss of excitatory input from the brain and inhibitory input below the level of the injury.

14. A primary assessment priority of a spinal-cord–injured patient is respiratory and airway status. One problem experienced in high-level cervical injuries is hypoventilation syndrome. A primary concern is that as the syndrome worsens the patient will experience respiratory arrest as he or she drops off to sleep. The patient experiences air hunger and is very anxious. Treatment for this syndrome includes

    A. high levels of oxygen to maintain the hypoxic drive

    B. antianxiety medications to assist easy respirations

    C. nighttime mechanical ventilation for about 10 days

    D. continuous ventilation until the syndrome subsides

Correct answer: C

Rationale: Nighttime ventilation is the treatment of choice. Caution is used with patients dependent on the hypoxic drive for breathing, continuous ventilation is not necessary, and antianxiety drugs might worsen the hypoventilation.

15. Patients with injuries above C5 have a decrease in or loss of sympathetic innervation. You would then expect to see which of the following responses?

    A. vasodilation

    B. vasoconstriction

    C. tachycardia

    D. hypertension

Correct answer: A

Rationale: Vasodilation, decreased venous return, hypotension, and bradycardia are effects of this loss of sympathetic outflow. The vasomotor response returns over the course of 1–3 months.

16. Autonomic dysreflexia is a problem that occurs in patients who have lesions above T6 after spinal shock has ceased. This problem can be life-threatening and ongoing. When the patient experiences this exaggerated sympathetic response to stimuli the nurse should first

    A. call the doctor

    B. elevate the head of the bed

    C. find the cause and remove it

    D. call for help

Correct answer: B

Rationale: The head of the bed should be elevated to decrease the hypertension while looking for and removing the cause. The doctor need only be called for orders for medications if removal of the cause does not eliminate the severe hypertension.

17. Rupturing of a cerebral aneurysm is a common cause of cerebral bleeds. When these aneurysms rupture, they typically rupture into the

    A. ventricular system

    B. brain tissue

    C. parenchymal tissue

    D. subarachnoid space

Correct answer: D

Rationale: Cerebral aneurysms generally rupture into the subarachnoid space.

18. Vasospasm is a narrowing of arteries adjacent to an aneurysm, which results in ischemia and infarction of brain tissue if unresolved. The nurse must be alert to this potential problem and know that vasospasm usually occurs ____ to ____ days after a cerebral aneurysm rupture.

    A. 1–2

    B. 20–30

    C. 4–14

    D. there is no expected time period

Correct answer: C

Rationale: This usually occurs 4–14 days after aneurysm rupture.

19. Cerebral angiography is sometimes performed on patients with acute CVA. Nursing assessment of the patient who is to undergo angiography includes
    A. inspection for hematoma
    B. immobilization of patient
    C. circulatory checks
    D. baseline neurological assessment

Correct answer: D

Rationale: Baseline assessment is important before angiography.

20. Care of the patient with an hemorrhagic CVA would include
    A. dimming the room lights and turning down volume of patient's monitors
    B. providing medications such as anticonvulsants and antifibrinolytics
    C. providing bed rest and a quiet environment
    D. all of the above

Correct answer: D

Rationale: All of these actions are standard for a hemorrhagic CVA.

CASE STUDIES

CASE STUDY #1

Mr. M. is a 35-year-old married man who works construction. He is admitted due to involvement in a motor vehicle accident. He was riding a motorcycle that ran into the side of a van. He sustained multiple trauma and was unconscious at the scene. He apparently had no skull fractures but did have multiple facial fractures, including an open fracture of the frontal sinuses, sphenoid fracture, lateral wall of the orbit fracture, and deviated nasal septum, which was a zygomatic fracture. His original CAT scan of the head was negative for fracture and hemorrhage. As he gradually woke up, however, it became apparent that he had posttraumatic amnesia and was having definite cognitive and judgment problems. It was later determined that he had developed epidural and subdural hematoma, which were surgically removed. He also had a tracheostomy, which has been removed.

1. Due to his injury and subsequent surgery, the nurse would be concerned about potential altered cerebral tissue perfusion. What are the goals for this problem?

    Having mean arterial pressure range of 63–124 mmHg, systolic BP 100–140 mmHg, diastolic range of 60–90 mmHg, stable VS, urine output >/= 30 ml/hr, H&H WNL, normal sinus rhythm, CVP 3–10 mmHg, PCWP 5–15 mmHg, improved neurological status, ABGs WNL.

2. What are the nursing interventions for this patient?

    Make a neurological assessment every hour; monitor BP and pulse every hour; monitor correlation between BP and neurological status; monitor respiratory status; monitor ECG pattern continuously; check CVP and PAP as ordered; monitor urine output hourly and specific gravity every two hours; check for hematuria; assess for signs of bleeding from chest, abdomen, pelvis, and extremities; provide a calm, quiet environment; monitor effect of administered medications such as heparin and warfarin; administer medications for vasospasm; minimize restlessness and agitation; monitor electrolytes, H&H, serum osmolality, and ABGs.

3. The nurse should teach Mr. M. and his family about which complication of head injury?

    Seizures

4. What are some important points that the nurse should explain to Mr. M.?

    The most important point is that antiseizure medication should not be stopped without consulting the physician. The nurse should also teach specific side effects of the designated medication. The patient and family need to know safety measures to take in the event of a seizure.

CASE STUDY #2

Ms. F., a 22-year-old unmarried college student, is injured while surfing. She is diagnosed with complete C6 spinal cord injury.

1. What problems would the nurse expect in the early phase of Ms. F.'s care?

    Respiratory status, pulmonary emboli, stress ulcers, autonomic dysreflexia, maintenance of alignment, maintenance of vital signs, paralytic ileus, urinary incontinence, expressed concerns of long-term deficits (i.e., walking).

2. Long-term concerns would involve what types of needs?

    Mobility, self care, bowel and bladder control, self worth, nutritional requirements.

3. Describe the goals and related nursing interventions for one long-term concern, such as nutritional status.

    Goals: bowel sounds present, absence of abdominal distention, absence of vomiting, potassium WNL, absence of T-wave depression, gastric secretions and stool negative for occult blood, maintain gastric pH > 3, H&H WNL, maintain admission weight, return of bowel movements and flatus.

    Nursing interventions: use of NG tube on low suction to prevent abdominal distention and possible aspiration, daily weights with bed scale, measure abdominal girths every 8–72 hours, NPO until bowel sounds present, nutritional assessment, parenteral hyperalimentation if ordered, advance diet slowly (start with clear liquids in small amounts and increase as tolerated), monitor serum albumin and proteins initially and every three days thereafter, monitor gastric pH of NG tube, aspirate, administer antacids and H_2 receptor blockers, note that sudden unexplained shoulder pain can be referred pain from GI tract.

4. Ms. F. tells the nurse she wants to die. What kind of response should the nurse make?

    The nurse should use therapeutic techniques to encourage further verbalization of concerns, offer hope without dishonesty as to potential for future.

Chapter 10 Case Studies

CASE STUDY #1

Mr. M. is a 35-year-old married man who works construction. He is admitted due to involvement in a motor vehicle accident. He was riding a motorcycle that ran into the side of a van. He sustained multiple trauma and was unconscious at the scene. He apparently had no skull fractures but did have multiple facial fractures, including an open fracture of the frontal sinuses, sphenoid fracture, lateral wall of the orbit fracture, and deviated nasal septum, which was a zygomatic fracture. His original CAT scan of the head was negative for fracture and hemorrhage. As he gradually woke up, however, it became apparent that he had post-traumatic amnesia and was having definite cognitive and judgment problems. It was later determined that he had developed epidural and subdural hematoma, which were surgically removed. He also had a tracheostomy, which has been removed.

1. Due to his injury and subsequent surgery, the nurse would be concerned about potential altered cerebral tissue perfusion. What are the goals for this problem?

2. What are the nursing interventions for this patient?

3. The nurse should teach Mr. M. and his family about which complication of head injury?

4. What are some important points that the nurse should explain to Mr. M.?

Chapter 10 Case Studies

CASE STUDY #2

Ms. F., a 22-year-old unmarried college student, is injured while surfing. She is diagnosed with complete C6 spinal cord injury.

1. What problems would the nurse expect in the early phase of Ms. F.'s care?

2. Long-term concerns would involve what types of needs?

3. Describe the goals and related nursing interventions for one long-term concern, such as nutritional status.

4. Ms. F. tells the nurse she wants to die. What kind of response should the nurse make?

Pathophysiology Flow Diagram—Head Injury
Primary Injury (Acceleration-Deceleration Injury; Penetrating Injury)

Brain set into motion inside skull

(a) Structural changes in neurons (shearing, stretching, rotational, tearing forces)

{s/s—altered mentation, motor sensory, cranial nerve & autonomic function}

(b) Biochemical changes in neuron
Ca^{++} influx $-->$ ↑ free O_2 radicals
↑ Glutamate
↑ Lactate

Breakdown lipid neuronal membrane

Epidural/subdural hematoma

(c) Vascular changes

Loss of autoregulation

↓ Cerebral blood flow $-->$ cerebral edema $-->$ ICP

Ischemia $-->$ IICP

Infarction {s/s—permanent neurological dysfunction}

Damage to neurons/pathways

Secondary Brain Injury

(a) Increased brain tissue, CSF, blood from primary injury

↓ Compliance

IICP

(b) Loss of cerebral autoregulation
↓ Cerebral blood flow $-->$ Impaired chemical regulation
↓ PO_2, ↑ PCO_2, $-->$ hypoxia
↓ ATP $-->$ ↓ Na-K pump $-->$ Cerebral edema

Ischemia

Infarction

IICP

Skull Fracture

Outbending of skull
Moves toward point of impact to base of skull   {s/s—headache, stunned}

(a) Linear Skull Fx

Fx floor of cranial vault

Torn dura $-->$ {s/s—CSF leak, headache photophobia, nuchal rigidity}

Stretching neurons $-->$ {s/s—altered LOC, cranial nerve defects, motor & sensory dysfunction}

Soft tissue injury $-->$ {s/s—Raccoon eyes, periorbital edema, Battle signs}

(b) Basilar Skull Fx

Outer table depressed below inner table

Torn dura $-->$ {s/s—CSF leak, headache photophobia, nuchal rigidity}

Compressed brain tissue $-->$ below depressed bone   {altered consciousness, impaired motor & sensory function, impaired cranial nerve function}

(c) Depressed Skull Fx

DIRECTIONS

Diagram (draw) arrows demonstrating pathophysiology.

Table 10–9. DRUG THERAPY IN PATIENTS WITH INCREASED INTRACRANIAL PRESSURE, HEAD INJURY, CEREBROVASCULAR ACCIDENT, SPINAL CORD INJURY, OR STATUS EPILEPTICUS

Drug	Actions/Uses	Dosage/Route	Side Effects	Nursing Implications
Mannitol (20%)	Draws water from normal brain cells into plasma; reduces ICP; increases CPP	1.5–2 g/kg initial IV over 0.5–1.0 hr then 0.25–0.5 g/kg IV every 3–5 hr depending on ICP, CPP, serum osmolality	Hypotension, dehydration, electrolyte imbalance, tachycardia, rebound edema	1–2 hr neurological assessments; monitor ICP, CPP, serum osmolality; hourly I&O; daily weights, monitor electrolytes, monitor ABGs, VS
Furosemide (Lasix)	Renal tubular diuretic; reduces cerebral edema by drawing sodium and water out of injured neurons; decreases CSF production	1 mg/kg IV bolus every 6–12 hr (Becker and Gudeman, 1989)	Ototoxicity, polyuria, electrolyte disturbances, gastric irritation, muscle cramps, hypotension	Same as above
Dexamethasone (Decadron)	Steroid that has a stabilizing effect on cell membrane and prevents destructive effect of free O_2 radicals; decreases inflammation by suppressing white cells	6–20 mg IV initial then 4–6 mg every 6 hr IV	Flushing, sweating, hypotension, tachycardia, thrombocytopenia, weakness, nausea, diarrhea, GI irritation/hemorrhage, fluid retention, poor wound healing, weight gain	Decreases effects of anticoagulants, anticonvulsants, antidiabetic agents; increases effects of digitalis; monitor glucose, potassium, daily weights; monitor VS; causes edema; taper drug prior to discontinuing
Cimetidine	Inhibits histamine at the H_2 receptor sites, inhibiting gastric acid secretion; decreases GI irritation to stress response following neurological injury and steroid use	300 mg in 50 ml 0.9% NaCl every 6–8 hr	Diarrhea, increases BUN, creatinine, thrombocytopenia; increases prothrombin time, bradycardia	Increases toxicity of phenytoin, lidocaine, procainamide; antacids decrease action of cimetidine; give slowly IV—can cause bradycardia

Drug	Action	Dose	Side Effects	Nursing Considerations
Labetalol	Beta-blocker that is nonselecting; decreases blood pressure	200 mg in 200 ml 0.9% NS at 2 mg/min IV; repeat every 6–8 hr as needed or 20 mg/over 2 min IV bolus; may repeat 40–80 mg every 10 min not to exceed 300 mg (Skidmore-Roth, 1988)	Hypotension, bradycardia, CHF, ventricular dysrhythmias, drowsiness, lethargy, nausea, tinnitis, wheezing	Cimetidine increases hypotension; increases hypoglycemia; hourly I&O; daily weights; monitor BP, pulse; taper drug if long-term use
Phenytoin (Dilantin)	Inhibits the spread of seizures; SE	For SE, 10–15 mg/kg loading dose IV not to exceed a rate of 50 mg/min; can be infused mixed with NS at doses of 20 mg/kg, rate not to exceed 50 mg/min	Bradycardia, hypotension nystagmus/ataxia—dose-related gingival hyperplasia, blood dyscrasias; rash	Slow rate down if bradycardia or cardiac arrhythmias occur; monitor ECG and BP; monitor lab; monitor respiratory status
Diazepam (Valium)	Depresses subcortical areas of CNS; SE	5–10 mg initially; may be repeated at 10- to 15-min intervals up to a maximum of 30 mg, rate of administration not to exceed 2 mg/min	Respiratory depression, hypotension, drowsiness, dry mouth	Monitor respiratory status; administer IV bolus in a large vein
Lorazepam (Ativan)	Same as diazepam	2–4 mg IV bolus	Respiratory depression, hypotension, drowsiness	Same as diazepam
Pentobarbital	Sedation; barbiturate metabolism and energy requirements; may prevent peroxidation of lipid components of cell membrane; used for refractory increased ICP and refractory SE	For increased ICP: 3–5 mg/kg IV in boluses of 50–100 mg doses monitoring ICP—loading dose; hourly maintenance doses of 100–200 mg (1–2 mg/kg) For SE: 2–8 mg/kg IV loading dose; maintenance dose 1–3 mg/kg/hr IV	Hypotension (at time of bolus), myocardial depression; respiratory depression	Monitor ICP (goal is to decrease ICP 15–20 mm Hg), monitor CPP; monitor vital signs and hemodynamic status, response of individual patients is variable; each one must be monitored closely

Table 10–3. MECHANISMS OF CLOSED HEAD INJURY WITH ASSOCIATED SIGNS/SYMPTOMS—IMPACT SETS BRAIN INTO MOTION INSIDE RIGID SKULL

Injury	Signs and Symptoms
Skull Fractures (Deformation of Skull, Secondary to Impact)	
Linear: Starts at outbended area, moves toward point of impact and to base of skull	Swelling, redness, bruising, tenderness on scalp, scalp laceration
Depressed: Outer table depressed below the inner table, associated with torn dura, and brain beneath depressed bone is bruised	Palpation of depressed area in contour of skull; CSF leak from nose, ear, postnasal; scalp bruising, tenderness, laceration
Basilar: Fracture is the anterior, middle, and/or posterior fossa along the floor of the cranial vault, dura is torn	
Anterior Fossa Fracture	Raccoon or panda eyes, periorbital edema, CSF leak nose, nasal congestion, cranial nerve deficits
Middle Fossa Facture	CSF leak ear, hematympanum, battle sign, decreased hearing, cranial nerve deficits
Posterior Fossa Fracture	Bruising base of the neck, cranial nerve deficits
Cellular Injuries to Brain Cells (Interruption of Normal Connections, Neurons, Pathways; Biochemical Changes Secondary to Stretching, Shearing, Rotational and Shearing Forces Associated with Impact)	
Focal Injuries: Concussion, contusion, avulsion	
Concussion: Altered LOC, confusion, disorientation, retrograde amnesia	
Contusion: Injury can be to the area directly beneath impact (coup) or injury can be to the brain's poles (contrecoup); since these areas are prone to bleeding and swelling, they act as an intracranial expanding mass	Altered level of consciousness, retrograde amnesia, motor deficits (weakness to paralysis), restlessness, combative, confusion, speech disturbances, cranial nerve dysfunction, decorticate and decerebrate posturing, abnormal breathing patterns, coma
Penetrating Injuries: Injury is caused by deep laceration of brain tissue, damage to the ventricular system	
Low Velocity: Stab wound—injury is caused by deep laceration of brain tissue, damage to the ventricular system	
High Velocity: Gunshot wound—extensive injury because of the entry of many bone fragments at the site, bullets spin irregularly creating many paths, increasing the brain damage, and shock waves cause brain disruption	
Diffuse Brain Injury: Tearing of axons and myelin sheaths, secondary to generalized movement of brain from impact—prolonged coma, cranial nerve deficits, motor deficits	
Secondary Injury: Caused by increased ICP, cerebral edema, herniation, ischemia, hypoxia; these situations complicate intracerebral bleeds, focal and penetrating injuries	Prolonged coma, cranial nerve deficits, motor deficits
Intracerebral Bleeds (Cerebral Vessels Are Broken or Sheared Off Secondary to Impact)	
Epidural: Tearing of an artery from a skull fracture, brisk bleeding and rapid accumulation in the epidural space	Onset short period of LOC then lucid, then confusion, irritability, headache, deterioration LOC, motor, CN
Subdural: Tearing of bridging cortical veins—blood accumulates in the space between the dura and arachnoid	Acute and subacute—depressed LOC, pupil and extraocular movement changes, motor changes; headache, *chronic* personality changes, gait problems
Subarachnoid: Bleeding into the subarachnoid space from the rupture of a traumatic aneurysm; altered LOC, headache, nuchal rigidity, photophobia	
Intraventricular: Bleeding to the ventricles; altered LOC, cranial nerve dysfunction, motor changes	
Intracerebral: Bleeding into brain tissue, producing necrosis	Similar to focal injuries

Table 10–1. THE 12 CRANIAL NERVES

Cranial Nerve	Name	Major Functions
I	Olfactory	Smell
II	Optic	Vision
III	Oculomotor	Movements of eyes; pupillary constriction and accommodation
IV	Trochlear	Movement of eyes
V	Trigeminal	Muscles of mastication and eardrum tension; general sensations from anterior half of head, including face, nose, mouth, and meninges
VI	Abducens	Movements of eyes
VII	Facial	Muscles of facial expression and tension on ear bones (stapes); lacrimination and salivation; taste
VIII	Auditory	Hearing and equilibrium reception (vestibulocochlear)
IX	Glossopharyngeal	Swallowing; salivation; taste; visceral sensory
X	Vagus	Swallowing movements and laryngeal control; parasympathetics to thoracic and abdominal viscera
XI	Spinal accessory	Movements of head and shoulders
XII	Hypoglossal	Movements of tongue

From Marshall, S. B., et al. (1990). *Neuroscience critical care.* Philadelphia: W. B. Saunders Co.

Table 10–4. SPINAL NERVE INNERVATION OF MAJOR MUSCLE GROUPS

Spinal Nerve	Muscle Group Movement	Assessment Technique
C4–C5	Shoulder abduction	Shrug shoulders against downward pressure of examiner's hands
C5–C6	Elbow flexion (biceps)	Arm is pulled up from resting position against resistance
C7	Elbow extension (triceps)	From the flexed position, arm is straightened out against resistance
C7	Thumb-index pinch	Index finger is held firmly to thumb against resistance to pull apart
C8	Hand grasp	Hand grasp strength is evaluated
L2–L4	Hip flexion	Leg is lifted from bed against resistance
L5–S1	Knee flexion	Knee is flexed against resistance
L2–L4	Knee extension	From flexed position, knee is extended against resistance
L5	Foot dorsiflexion	Foot pulled up toward nose against resistance
S1	Foot plantar flexion	Foot pushed down (stepping on the gas) against resistance

From Marshall, S. B., et al. (1990). *Neuroscience critical care*. Philadelphia: W. B. Saunders Co.

Acute Respiratory Failure

TERMINOLOGY

- Acute
- Adult respiratory distress syndrome (ARDS)
- Alveolar ventilation
- Asthma
- Atelectasis
- "Bucking" ventilator
- Chronic
- Chronic bronchitis
- Chronic obstructive pulmonary disease (COPD)
- Dead space
- Deep vein thrombosis (DVT)
- Diffusion defect
- Dyspnea
- Emphysema

- Hemoptysis
- Hypercapnia
- Hypocarbia
- Hypoxemia
- Hypoxia
- Intrapulmonary shunting
- Minute ventilation
- Neuromuscular blocking agent
- Pneumoconstriction
- Pulmonary toilet
- Pulmonary embolus (PE)
- Respiratory failure
- Surfactant
- Ventilation-perfusion mismatching

OUTLINE

I. Acute respiratory failure
    A. Definition

    B. Pathophysiology

      1. Failure of oxygenation

        a. Hypoventilation

          1. Definition

          2. Causes

3. Treatment

  b. Intrapulmonary shunting

    1. Definition

    2. Shunt estimation

  c. Ventilation/perfusion mismatching

    1. Definition

  d. Diffusion defects

    1. Definition

    2. Causes

  e. Low cardiac output

    1. Definition

    2. Effects on oxygenation

  f. Low hemoglobin

    1. Definition

    2. Effects on oxygenation

  g. Tissue hypoxia

    1. Anaerobic metabolism

    2. Signs and symptoms

2. Failure of ventilation

  a. Hypoventilation

    1. Definition

    2. Causes

  b. Ventilation-perfusion mismatching

    1. Dead space

    2. Signs and symptoms

II. Adult respiratory distress syndrome (ARDS)
  A. Definition

  B. Etiology

    1. Risk factors

    2. Mortality rate

  C. Pathophysiology

    1. Initial injury

      a. Alveolar capillary membrane changes

    2. Alveolar collapse

    3. Interstitial edema

    4. Intrapulmonary shunting

    5. Compensatory responses

    6. O_2 toxicity

  D. Assessment

    1. Timing of early symptoms

    2. Initial signs

      a. Change behavior

      b. Dyspnea/hyperventilation

      c. Respiratory alkalosis

    d. Increased peak inspiratory pressure

    e. Increased pulse

    f. Increased temperature

  3. Progression of process

      a. Severe dyspnea

      b. Decreased paO_2—hypoxemia

      c. Decreased $paCO_2$—respiratory alkalosis

      d. Tachycardia

      e. Pallor/cyanosis

  4. Metabolic acidosis

  5. Changing pulmonary mechanics

  6. Key clinical findings

E. Nursing diagnoses

  1. Goals

      a. Increase delivery of O_2 to tissues

      b. Decrease overall O_2 consumption

      c. Supply nutrition to meet metabolic demands

      d. Maintain fluid and electrolyte balance

      e. Support patient and family

  2. List

      a. Ineffective breathing pattern

      b. Impaired gas exchange

    c. High risk for infection

    d. Fluid volume excess

    e. Altered nutrition: less than body requirements

    f. High risk for impaired skin integrity

    g. Altered tissue perfusion: cardiopulmonary

    h. Altered tissue perfusion: peripheral

    i. Potential anxiety

    j. High risk for ineffective family coping

    k. Activity intolerance

F. Interventions

  1. Oxygenation

      a. Mechanical ventilation

        1. "Bucking"

        2. Monitoring lines

        3. Effects on hemodynamics

            a. Cardiac output

            b. Peripheral circulation

        4. Pulmonary hygiene

      b. Decreased O_2 consumption

        2. Fluid and electrolyte balance

            a. Volume replacement

                i.   Assessment

ii.   Crystalloids and colloids

3. Nutrition

4. Psychosocial support

5. Other therapies

G. Outcomes

1. Effective breathing pattern/adequate gas

2. Adequate oxygenation

3. Decreased O_2 consumption

4. Normothermic

5. Absence of infection

6. Optimal fluid balance

7. Adequate nutrition

8. Intact skin

9. Minimal damaage to lung tissue

10. Stable BP and CO

11. Decreased anxiety

12. Gradual increase in activity

III. Chronic obstructive pulmonary disease (COPD)
A. Definition

B. Pathophysiology

1. Asthma

a. Definition

b. Lung effects

c. Status asthmaticus

2. Emphysema

a. Definition

b. Lung effects

c. Cor pulmonale

d. Classic description

3. Chronic bronchitis

a. Definition

b. Lung effects

c. Classic description

C. Assessment

1. Baseline respiratory status

2. Arterial blood gasses (ABGs)

D. Nursing diagnosis

1. See ARDS

2. Decisional conflict

E. Interventions

1. Goals

a. Sustain during acute episode of failure

b. Return to previous level of functioning

2. Positioning

3. O_2 therapy

IV. Pulmonary embolism (PE)
  A. Definition

    1. Origin

    2. Types

  B. Etiology

    1. Virchow's Triad

      a. Venous stasis

      b. Disease state that alters blood coagulability

      c. Damage to vessel walls

  C. Pathophysiology

    1. Pulmonary

      a. Perfusion

      b. Pneumoconstriction

      c. Surfactant production

      d. Serotonin release

      e. Pulmonary hypertension

        1. Definition

        2. Signs and symptoms

        3. J receptors

      f. Infarct

    2. Prognosis

D. Assessment

  1. Risk factors

  2. Chief complaint

    a. Dyspnea

    b. Chest pain

  3. Medical-surgical history

  4. Cardiopulmonary

  5. Patient affect

  6. Lab tests

  7. Diagnostic studies

    a. Chest x-ray

    b. Ventilation-perfusion scan

    c. Pulmonary angiogram

E. Nursing diagnoses

  1. Goals

    a. Prevent further decreased O_2 to tissues

    b. Provide cardiopulmonary support

    c. Maintain fluid balance

    d. Support patient and family

  2. List

    a. Activity intolerance

    b. Anxiety

c. Decreased CO

d. High risk for ineffective family coping

e. Impaired gas exchange

f. High risk for fluid volume excess

g. High risk for injury

h. High risk for pain

i. Altered cardiopulmonary tissue perfusion

F. Interventions

  1. Prevention

  2. Hypoxemia/hypoxia

    a. Assessment

    b. Nursing interventions

  3. Chronic heart failure (CHF) potential

  4. Pain

  5. Nutrition

  6. Heparin therapy

  7. Thrombolytics

8. Surgery

G. Outcomes

  1. Increased activity

  2. No signs of apprehension

  3. Stable fluid balance

  4. Stable hemodynamics

  5. Stable cardiac rhythm

  6. Family members comfortable

  7. Adequate oxygen delivery

  8. Normal respiration

  9. Normal breath sounds

  10. pO_2 greater than 80%

  11. No edema

  12. No extension of clot

  13. PT and PTT therapeutic

  14. Relief of pain

  15. Adequate tissue perfusion

MULTIPLE CHOICE

1. Reduced arterial oxygen concentration is called
   A. hypoxia
   B. hypoventilation
   C. hypoxemia
   D. hypocarbia

Correct answer: C

Rationale: Hypoxemia refers to decreased oxygen in the blood.

2. An intrapulmonary shunt occurs with
   A. inadequate ventilation
   B. inadequate perfusion
   C. inadequate circulation
   D. inadequate secretion

Correct answer: A

Rationale: Intrapulmonary shunting occurs when areas of the lung are inadequately ventilated but adequately perfused.

3. As diffusion capacity is reduced, _____ is the first affected.
   A. $PaCO_2$
   B. PaO_2
   C. pH
   D. N

Correct answer: B

Rationale: CO_2 diffuses more readily than O_2, so hypoxemia results first.

4. One of the initial signs of hypoxia in the cardiovascular system is
   A. hypotension
   B. bradycardia
   C. failure
   D. tachycardia

Correct answer: D

Rationale: Tachycardia and mild hypertension may be initial signs of hypoxia in the CV system.

5. Anatomical dead space is normally ___% of the inspired volume.
   A. 10–20
   B. 25–30
   C. 40–50
   D. 3–5

Correct answer: B

Rationale: The lower and upper airways do not play a part in gas exchange, this is normally 25–30% of the inspired volume.

6. Early warning signs of ARDS include
   A. hyperventilation
   B. respiratory acidosis
   C. decreased PIP
   D. bradycardia

Correct answer: A

Rationale: Early warning signs include tachycardia, increased PIP, respiratory alkalosis, and hyperventilation.

7. In ARDS, atelectasis develops because of a decreased production of surfactant. Atelectasis means that alveoli are
   A. filled with fluid
   B. distended
   C. collapsed
   D. filled with protein

Correct answer: C

Rationale: Alveolar walls become unstable and collapse when the Type II pneumocytes do not produce surfactant.

8. Fluid leaking into the alveolar interstitial spaces causes
   A. alveolar expansion
   B. increased lung volume
   C. increased functional residual (FRC) capacity
   D. compression

Correct answer: D

Rationale: Alveolar collapse, decreased FRC, decreased lung volume, and compression are a result of interstitial edema.

9. The V/Q mismatch and hypoxemia resulting from intrapulmonary shunting cause
   A. increased compliance
   B. hypoventilation
   C. hypocapnia
   D. decreased airway resistance

Correct answer: C

Rationale: Hypocapnia results from tachypnea as the patient tries to increase his or her PaO_2.

10. Tracheobronchitis, cough, inspiratory pain, and dyspnea are initial symptoms of
    A. PE
    B. pneumonia
    C. ARDS
    D. O_2 toxicity

Correct answer: D

Rationale: When levels of O_2 greater than 50% are utilized for an extended period of time, O_2 toxicity may result.

11. Your patient's ABGs indicate hypoxemia. The first intervention to relieve hypoxemia is
    A. supplemental O_2
    B. endotracheal suctioning
    C. positive end expiratory pressure (PEEP)
    D. high tidal volume

Correct answer: A

Rationale: The first intervention to attempt to relieve hypoxemia is to supply supplemental oxygen.

12. A paradoxical decrease in O_2 delivery may occur with PEEP. For this reason, the nurse should monitor
    A. heart rate
    B. blood pressure
    C. respiratory rate
    D. mentation

Correct answer: B

Rationale: The increase in pleural pressure with PEEP may result in decrease venous return which will decrease CO and BP, causing a decrease in O_2 delivery.

13. In unilateral disease, gas exchange may improve by positioning the patient with the good lung down. This occurs because
    A. there is better blood flow to the good lung
    B. the good lung expands more easily
    C. healing occurs more quickly in the diseased lung
    D. the diseased lung inflates more easily

Correct answer: A

Rationale: Increased blood flow to the better-functioning lung results in improved gas exchange.

14. Asthmatic patients' lungs become overinflated and stiff. This increases the work of breathing and results in
    A. bradypnea
    B. hypoventilation
    C. decreased pH
    D. decreased $PaCO_2$

Correct answer: D

Rationale: Increased work of breathing results in tachypnea, hyperventilation, and decreased $PaCO_2$.

15. Right-sided heart failure in response to elevated pulmonary artery pressure is called
    A. cardiogenic pulmonary edema
    B. cor pulmonale
    C. emphysema
    D. noncardiogenic pulmonary edema

Correct answer: B

Rationale: Cor pulmonale may occur as the right ventricle dilates and hypertrophies in response to elevated pulmonary artery pressure.

16. Baseline ABGs for a COPD patient might show
    A. PaO_2 75 and CO_2 40
    B. PaO_2 50 and $PaCO_2$ 35
    C. PaO_2 55 and $PaCO_2$ 55
    D. PaO_2 70 and $PaCO_2$ 50

Correct answer: C

Rationale: A COPD patient who chronically retains CO_2 may have baseline ABGs that show both PaO_2 and $PaCO_2$ in the 50–59 mmHg range.

17. Breathing as a result of the hypoxic drive means breathing in response to
    A. increased pH
    B. increased CO_2
    C. decreased O_2
    D. decreased pH

Correct answer: C

Rationale: Patients who normally return CO_2 breathe as a result of low PaO_2.

18. Virchow's Triad refers to
    A. the syndrome of ARDS
    B. mechanisms which identify tamponade
    C. the syndrome of CHF
    D. mechanisms that favor development of thrombi

Correct answer: D

Rationale: Vichow's Triad includes: 1) venous stasis; 2) disease states that alter coagulability; and 3) damage to the vessel walls.

19. Most frequently, the chief complaint of a patient with a PE is
    A. pain
    B. hemoptysis
    C. palpitation
    D. breathlessness

Correct answer: D

Rationale: Sudden onset of dyspnea or breathlessness is most frequently seen in PE patients.

20. One of the earliest signs of hypoxemia is
    A. tachypnea
    B. restlessness
    C. tachycardia
    D. cyanosis

Correct answer: B

Rationale: Restlessness, an early indicator of hypoxemia, should prompt the nurse to perform a more detailed assessment.

CASE STUDIES

CASE STUDY #1

Ms. J. had a cholecystectomy two days ago. She has resisted all attempts to move. She recently gave birth to a baby girl and has been on oral contraceptives for the last two years. She is overweight and has a sedentary lifestyle. After visiting hours are over, she complains of sudden onset of chest pain and becomes short of breath and apprehensive. Further assessment reveals a warm, red, tender right calf that is larger in circumference than the left. Considering her history and present signs and symptoms, a diagnosis of pulmonary embolism (PE) is made.

1. What diagnostic study will make the differential diagnosis?

   Pulmonary angiography

2. What is the underlying pathophysiology that causes impaired gas exchange in PE?

   Ventilation-perfusion imbalance
   Pneumoconstriction
   Atelectasis

3. Name Ms. J's risk factors for PE.

   Recent surgery
   Immobility
   Overweight
   Oral contraceptives
   Deep vein thrombosis (DVT)

Ms. J. is given supplemental O_2 and morphine for pain relief. After a bolus dose of heparin, she is started on a continuous infusion at 1000 units/hr.

4. What lab values are used to determine heparin dosing?

   Partial thromboplastin time (PTT)

5. Planning Ms. J's care means looking ahead to discharge. What health teaching will she require?

   Drugs
   Diet
   Activity
   Wound care

CASE STUDY #2

Mr. S., a 24-year-old accountant, was involved in a motor vehicle accident in which he sustained a fractured pelvis and left femur with crush injuries to his lower left leg. He was fluid resuscitated because of hypotension. In the 24 hours following his admission, he became increasingly restless and apprehensive. His chest x-ray was clear and he was mildly alkalotic. He rapidly became dyspneic, his lungs noisy, and his ABGs deteriorated even though his supplemental O_2 was increased from a nasal cannula to a nonrebreather face mask. He was intubated and placed on mechanical ventilation with a high concentration of O_2 and PEEP. His subsequent chest x-ray showed pulmonary infiltrates and consolidation. He was diagnosed as having noncardiogenic pulmonary edema.

1. Why is ARDS described as noncardiogenic pulmonary edema?

    Pulmonary edema develops not from left ventricular failure but because of a primary event that usually involves a period of hypotension, which results in lung insult.

2. What is the hallmark sign of ARDS? Describe this in Mr. S.'s case.

    Refractory hypoxemia is the hallmark of ARDS. Mr. S.'s supplemental O_2 was increased from a nasal cannula to a nonrebreather mask without increasing his pO_2.

3. How does PEEP affect ARDS?

    PEEP maintains positive pressure in airways at all times, keeping alveolar sacs inflated and decreasing venous return.

4. Is dyspnea subjective or objective? Why?

    Subjective: it is the sensation experienced by the patient as fluid moves from pulmonary capillaries to alveolar interstitial space.

5. Name some options for communicating with Mr. S.

    Lip reading
    Helping him to write messages
    Writing messages for him
    Pointing to letter/picture board

Chapter 11 Case Studies

CASE STUDY #1

Ms. J. had a cholecystectomy two days ago. She has resisted all attempts to move. She recently gave birth to a baby girl and has been on oral contraceptives for the last two years. She is overweight and has a sedentary lifestyle. After visiting hours are over, she complains of sudden onset of chest pain and becomes short of breath and apprehensive. Further assessment reveals a warm, red, tender right calf that is larger in circumference than the left. Considering her history and present signs and symptoms, a diagnosis of pulmonary embolism (PE) is made.

1. What diagnostic study will make the differential diagnosis?

2. What is the underlying pathophysiology that causes impaired gas exchange in PE?

3. Name Ms. J.'s risk factors for PE.

Ms. J. is given supplemental O_2 and morphine for pain relief. After a bolus dose of heparin, she is started on a continuous infusion at 1000 units/hr.

4. What lab values are used to determine heparin dosing?

5. Planning Ms. J.'s care means looking ahead to discharge. What health teaching will she require?

Chapter 11 Case Studies

CASE STUDY #2

Mr. S., a 24-year-old accountant, was involved in a motor vehicle accident in which he sustained a fractured pelvis and left femur with crush injuries to his lower left leg. He was fluid resuscitated because of hypotension. In the 24 hours following his admission, he became increasingly restless and apprehensive. His chest x-ray was clear and he was mildly alkalotic. He rapidly became dyspneic, his lungs noisy, and his ABGs deteriorated even though his supplemental O_2 was increased from a nasal cannula to a nonrebreather face mask. He was intubated and placed on mechanical ventilation with a high concentration of O_2 and PEEP. His subsequent chest x-ray showed pulmonary infiltrates and consolidation. He was diagnosed as having noncardiogenic pulmonary edema.

1. Why is ARDS described as noncardiogenic pulmonary edema?

2. What is the hallmark sign of ARDS? Describe this in Mr. S.'s case.

3. How does PEEP affect ARDS?

4. Is dyspnea subjective or objective? Why?

5. Name some options for communicating with Mr. S.

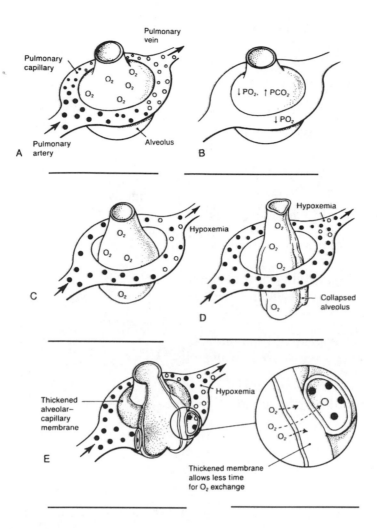

A — Pulmonary capillary; Pulmonary artery; Pulmonary vein; Alveolus; O_2

B — $\downarrow PO_2$, $\uparrow PCO_2$; $\downarrow PO_2$

C — O_2; Hypoxemia

D — Hypoxemia; Collapsed alveolus; O_2

E — Thickened alveolar–capillary membrane; Hypoxemia; O_2; Thickened membrane allows less time for O_2 exchange

_____

_____

_____

_____

_____

_____

DIRECTIONS

Label the causes of hypoxemia.

_____

Figure 11–1. The four physiological causes of hypoxemia. *A*, A normal alveolar-capillary unit. Unoxygenated blood (filled circles) in the pulmonary capillary obtains O_2 from the alveolus. Oxygenated blood (open circles) leaves via the pulmonary veins. *B*, Hypoventilation results in an increased PCO_2 and decreased PO_2. *C*, Ventilation/perfusion mismatch resulting from poor alveolar ventilation; hypoxemia results. *D*, Right-to-left shunt. Hypoxemia results from many disorders, all of which lead to collapsed alveoli. *E*, Diffusion defect. The diffusion of O_2 across the aveolar-capillary membrane is decreased when the membrane is thickened or filled with fluid. (From Yee, B. H., and Zorb, S. L.: Cardiac Critical Care Nursing. Boston, Little, Brown, 1985, Fig. 5–4, p. 109.)

Lung injury

Pulmonary hypoperfusion

Tissue hypoxia   Platelet and leukocyte

Lactic acidosis   Occlusion of pulmonary
                                  microcirculation due to
                                  intravascular clotting

Release of vasoactive substances
(serotonin, histamine, bradykinin)

| Tachypnea Dyspnea Tachycardia |

↑ Permeability of the alveolar
capillary membrane

| ↑ Tachypnea ↑ Dyspnea Cyanosis Hypoxemia |

↑ Leakage of fluid into the
interstitial space and alveoli

Noncardiogenic pulmonary edema

| ↓ Compliance Crackles (rales) Gurgles (ronchi) | Fluid-filled   Injury to the type II
                                  alveoli   pneumocytes

                                                          ↓ Surfactant | Thick, frothy sputum Hypoxemia Respiratory distress |

| ↑ Tachypnea ↑ Hypocapnea ↓ pH ↑ PaCO₂ ↓ PaO₂ ↓ HCO₃⁻ Confusion | ↓ Compliance   Atelectasis

                                  ↑ Hypoxemia

                                  ↓ FRC

| Key:
_____ Indicates progression of process if not corrected
_ _ _ _ Indicates signs and symptoms associated with physiological changes |

DIRECTIONS

Make the connections using the key at the bottom.

Figure 10–2. Pathophysiology of ARDS.

Chapter

12

Acute Renal Failure

TERMINOLOGY

- Acute renal failure
- Adenosinetriphosphate (ATP)
- Albumin
- Aluretic
- Ammonia
- Anthropometric
- Antiemetic
- Anuria
- Arteriovenous fistula
- Arteriovenous shunt
- Catabolism
- Chemotaxis
- Chvostek's sign
- Coagulopathy
- Computed tomography (CT scan)
- Creatinine
- Creatinine clearance
- Dialysate
- Dialysis
- Diffusion
- Disequilibrium syndrome

- Drybody weight
- Ecchymosis
- Erythropoietin
- Extracorporeal
- Filtration
- Glomerular filtration
- Guaiac
- Hematuria
- Hemodialysis
- Hemofiltration
- Integument
- Intravenous pyelography (IVP)
- Micturition
- Nephrosonography
- Nocturia
- Oliguria
- Osmosis
- Parenchymal renal failure
- Pericarditis
- Peritoneal dialysis
- Petechiae

- Phagocytosis
- Polyuria
- Postrenal failure
- Prerenal failure
- Renal angiography
- Pruritus
- Purpura
- Renal osteodystrophy
- Renin
- Stomatitis
- Syncope

- ■ Transferrin
- ■ Trousseau's sign
- ■ Ultrafiltration
- ■ Urea
- ■ Uremic encephalopathy
- ■ Uremic frost
- ■ Uremic halitosis
- ■ Uremic toxins
- ■ Urochrome
- ■ Viscera

OUTLINE

I. Introduction
   A. Occurrence

   B. Morbidity/mortality

II. Renal anatomy
   A. Position

   B. Nephron

   C. Blood supply

   D. Blood flow through kidney

III. Renal physiology
   A. Regulation of fluid and electrolytes and excretion of waste

      1. Filtration

      2. Glomerular filtration rate (GFR)

      3. Reabsorption

   4. Secretion

   B. Regulation of acid-base balance

      1. Bicarbonate

      2. Hydrogen ion (H+)

   C. Blood pressure regulation

      1. Juxtaglomerular apparatus (JGA)

      2. Renin-angiotensin-aldosterone cascade (RAAC)

IV. Acute renal failure
   A. Definition

   B. Etiology

      1. Prerenal

         a. Definition

         b. Causes

2. Postrenal

   a. Definition

   b. Causes

3. Intrinsic/intrarenal

   a. Definition

   b. Causes

C. Pathophysiology of acute tubular necrosis (ATN)

  1. Mechanisms of oliguria

    a. Renal vasoconstriction

    b. Cellular edema

    c. Decreased glomerular capillary permeability

    d. Intratubular obstruction

    e. Back leak glomerular filtrate

D. Course of ATN

  1. Initiation

  2. Maintenance

  3. Recovery

E. Assessment

  1. Patient history

  2. Vital signs

  3. Medication history

  4. Physical assessment

5. Lab values

   a. Serum values

   b. Urinary creatinine clearance

   c. Urine studies

    1. Urinalysis

    2. Electrolytes

    3. Specific gravity/osmolality

6. Noninvasive diagnostic procedures

   a. Intake and output (I&O)

   b. Weight

   c. X-rays

7. Invasive diagnostic procedures

F. Systemic manifestations

  1. Cardiovascular

    a. Volume

    b. Electrolytes

  2. Hematological

    a. Infection

    b. Anemia

  3. Respiratory

    a. Cough

    b. Volume

4. Gastrointestinal

    a. Caloric intake/catabolism

    b. Stomatitis

    c. GI bleeding

5. Neuromuscular

    a. EEG changes

    b. Cerebral edema

6. Psychosocial

    a. Altered mental processes

7. Integumentary

    a. Uremic yellowness

G. Nursing diagnoses

    1. Alteration fluid and electrolyte balance

    2. Alteration acid-base balance

    3. High risk infection

    4. Altered nutrition: less than

    5. High risk anxiety

    6. Knowledge deficit

H. Collaborative interventions

    1. Management of prerenal azotemia

        a. Treatment of hypovolemia

        b. Prevention

2. Management of postrenal azotemia

3. Management of intrinsic azotemia

    a. Prevention

        1. Goals

            a. Cardiovascular

            b. Volume

        2. Hydration

        3. Renal perfusion

        4. Antibiotic monitoring

    b. Infection

4. Drug therapy

    a. Diuretics

        1. Types

        2. Problems

    b. Dopamine

    c. Miscellaneous agents

    d. Considerations

        1. Dosage

        2. Effectiveness

            a. Peak

            b. Trough

        3. Dialysis

5. Dietary management

   a. Goal

   b. Recommendations

      1. Caloric intake

      2. Protein

      3. Sodium

      4. Potassium

      5. Calcium

      6. Fluid intake

   c. Total parenteral nutrition (TPN)

6. Management of fluid, electrolyte, and acid-base imbalances

   a. Fluid imbalance

   b. Electrolyte imbalance

      1. Treatment of hyperkalemia

      2. Treatment of hyponatremia

      3. Treatment of hypocalcemia

      4. Treatment of hyperphosphat–emia

      5. Treatment of hypermagnesemia

   c. Acid-base imbalance

      1. Metabolic acidosis

         a. Treatment

         b. Prevention of tetany

7. Dialysis therapy

   a. Definition

   b. Indications

   c. Principles and mechanisms

      1. Diffusion

      2. Ultrafiltration

   d. Vascular access

      1. Percutaneous venous catheters

      2. Arteriovenous (AV) fistula

      3. Arteriovenous graft

      4. External arteriovenous shunt

   e. Nursing care

      1. AV fistula/graft

      2. Percutaneous catheter

   f. Hemodialysis

      1. Definition

      2. Complications

         a. Hypotension

         b. Dysrhythmias

         c. Muscle cramps

         d. Decreased PaO_2

         e. Disequilibrium syndrome

f. Infection

g. Other, rarer complications

3. Care of patient

a. Monitor lab

b. Weight

c. Dialyzable medications

d. Antihypertensives

e. Assess vascular access

f. Assess after dialysis

G. Continuous renal replacement therapy

1. Indications

2. Advantages

3. Principles

a. Definition

b. Procedure

1. Factors that influence blood flow

4. Methods

a. Continuous arteriovenous hemofiltration (CAVH)

1. Indications

b. Continuous arteriovenous hemodialysis (CAVHD)

1. Indications

5. Complications

6. Nursing responsibilities

H. Peritoneal dialysis

1. Definition

2. Indications

3. Advantages

4. Disadvantages

5. Complications

a. Mechanical

b. Metabolic

c. Inflammatory reactions

6. Contraindications

I. Decision making: renal replacement therapy

J. Outcomes

1. Stable fluid balance

2. Body wieght within 2 lbs.

3. Stable vital signs

4. Normal skin turgor

5. Lab values and ABG within normal

6. Absence infection

7. Adequate nutrition

8. Patient and family participation in care

MULTIPLE CHOICE

1. The basic functional unit of the kidney is
   A. tubule
   B. renal corpuscle
   C. glomerulus
   D. nephron

Correct answer: D

Rationale: The nephron is the basic functional unit, composed of the renal corpuscle and tubule.

2. Glomerular filtration occurs due to
   A. a pressure gradient
   B. osmotic pressure
   C. filtration pressure
   D. hydrostatic pressure

Correct answer: A .

Rationale: A pressure gradient, the difference between forces that favor filtration and forces that oppose filtration, causes glomerular filtration.

3. Oliguria is defined as urine output
   A. less than 100 ml/24 hrs
   B. greater than 400 ml/24 hrs
   C. less than 400 ml/24 hrs
   D. less than 50 ml/24 hrs

Correct answer: C

Rationale: Anuria is urine output less than 100 ml/24 hrs; oliguria is less than 400 ml/24 hrs.

4. Prerenal failure is
   A. the period of time prior to frank failure
   B. failure caused by interference with renal perfusion
   C. the time before renal ischemia
   D. failure caused by obstruction

Correct answer: B

Rationale: Prerenal failure occurs because of poor renal perfusion such as decreased cardiac output, fluid volume loss, third spacing, and so on.

5. The most common cause of intrarenal failure is
   A. pyelonephritis
   B. renal calculi
   C. glomerulonephritis
   D. acute tubular necrosis (ATN)

Correct answer: D

Rationale: The most common cause of intrinsic azotemia is ATN, caused by prolonged ischemia or exposure to nephrotoxic agents.

6. ATN is potentially reversible in the
   A. maintenance phase
   B. recovery phase
   C. initiation phase
   D. convalescent phase

Correct answer: C

Rationale: During the initiation phase, from the primary event to the beginning of the change in urine output, ATN is potentially reversible.

7. An elevated blood urea nitrogen (BUN) may cause body temperature to be
   A. elevated
   B. subnormal
   C. normal
   D. labile

Correct answer: B

Rationale: An elevated BUN has an antipyretic effect.

8. Weight gain, edema, jugular vein distention (JVD), and increased BP in the presence of oliguria suggest what category of renal failure?
   A. intrinsic
   B. prerenal
   C. postrenal
   D. ischemic

Correct answer: A

Rationale: Oliguria with weight loss, decreased BP, tachycardia, flat neck veins, and poor skin turgor suggest a prerenal cause.

9. The best measure of renal function is
   A. urine output
   B. BUN
   C. urinary creatinine clearance
   D. urine electrolytes

Correct answer: C

Rationale: Because of creatinine's stability, variations in creatinine levels rapidly reflect changes in renal function.

10. Your patient's creatinine clearance is 5 ml/min. This data signifies
    A. normal renal function
    B. renal dysfunction
    C. inaccurate lab results
    D. hyperactive kidneys

Correct answer: B

Rationale: Normal creatinine clearance is 125 ml/min, so a value of 5 ml/min is consistent with renal dysfunction.

11. An elevated BUN may be caused by
    A. overhydration
    B. limited protein intake
    C. renal failure only
    D. corticosteroids

Correct answer: D

Rationale: There are extrarenal causes of an elevated BUN, which limits the test's ability to evaluate renal function.

12. Mr. K., a dialysis patient, gained 10 lb. since his last visit three days ago. Weight gain is attributed to fluid retention. You calculate that he retained
    A. 2 L
    B. 5000 cc
    C. 2600 cc
    D. 2400 cc

Correct answer: C

Rationale: There are approximately 500 cc/1 lb. and there is an 800 ml/24 insensible fluid loss.

$$cc = \left(\frac{500 \text{ cc} \times 10 \text{ lb.}}{1 \text{ lb.} \times 1} \right) - \frac{3 (800cc)}{\text{insensible loss}}$$

5000 cc – 2400 cc = 2600 cc

13. Acute renal failure (ARF) patients may have bleeding, hemolysis, decreased erythropoietin production hemodilution, and decreased erythrocyte survival time. All of these may cause
    A. anemia
    B. infection
    C. anorexia
    D. pneumonia

Correct answer: A

Rationale: Anemia can develop rapidly in ARF patients but it is usually mild.

14. Stomatitis associated with acute renal failure contributes to
    A. caloric wasting
    B. caloric excess
    C. tissue catabolism
    D. tissue anabolism

Correct answer: C

Rationale: Stomatitis inhibits the patient's ability to ingest food substances, increasing tissue catabolism.

15. Uremic yellowness is due to
    A. jaundice
    B. urochrome
    C. nitrogenous wastes
    D. bilirubin

Correct answer: B

Rationale: Urochrome pigment gives urine its yellow color. When urine output is down it seeks other excretory pathways.

16. Insertion of a ureteral stent would most likely be done for a patient with
    A. prerenal azotemia
    B. intrinsic azotemia
    C. postrenal azotemia
    D. intrarenal azotemia

Correct answer: C

Rationale: Postrenal obstruction may require a ureteral stent if the obstruction is due to calculi or carcinoma.

17. Two key goals in preventing intrinsic azotemia are maintenance of cardiovascular function and
    A. maintaining adequate intravascular volume
    B. decreasing tissue perfusion
    C. maintaining adequate cellular volume
    D. decreasing tissue edema

Correct answer: A

Rationale: These goals are accomplished by maintaining adequate hydration, maintaining renal perfusion, monitoring antibiotic administration, and weighing the risk/benefit ratio.

18. Because infection is life-threatening to renal failure patients, they should
    A. never be catheterized
    B. catheterized with a Foley
    C. have a catheter inserted immediately
    D. be catheterized intermittently

Correct answer: D

Rationale: If necessary, intermittent catheterization is preferable.

19. If a patient is being dialyzed, you may need to
    A. provide extra drug doses
    B. decrease drug doses
    C. give all drugs prior to dialysis
    D. give all drugs after dialysis

Correct answer: A

Rationale: Extra drug doses may be needed to avoid suboptimal drug levels.

20. Hyponatremia is generally the result of
    A. dehydration
    B. sodium excess
    C. water overload
    D. sodium deficit

Correct answer: C

Rationale: Sodium is measured in relation to water, so hyponatremia is often the result of water excess, which is treated with fluid restriction.

CASE STUDIES

CASE STUDY #1

Mr. G. is postop abdominal aortic aneurysm (AAA) repair. His hemodynamic status has stabilized but his urine output is low normal at best. Over the next hours, his urine output continues to fall. He develops bilateral crackles, a bounding pulse, and his BP and CVP rise. His BUN, creatinine, and K have also crept higher than his preop values.

1. Explain the reason for Mr. G.'s apparent renal failure.

   Acute tubular necrosis developed from renal ischemia during cross-clamping of the aorta for the AAA resection.

2. What do you expect to see as Mr. G. moves through the phases of acute tubular necrosis?

   Initiation phase—precipitating event to change urine output

   Maintenance phase—intrinsic renal damage has occurred, urine volume at lowest point

   Recovery phase—renal tissue recovers and repairs, urine output increases, lab values improve

3. What is the most sensitive indicator of renal function? Of renal perfusion? Why?

   Creatinine—nitrogenous waste from muscle metabolism, refers to renal function

   Urine output—refers to the body's ability to perfuse the kidneys

   Urine output may be normal or even elevated with concurrent renal dysfunction (i.e., the kidneys are being perfused but the glomeruli and/or the tubule cells are not functioning properly).

4. Mr. G. needs renal replacement therapy for his fluid overload, hyperkalemia, and acidotic state. How would you determine which therapy is suitable? Give reasons for each.

   Hemodialysis—Mr. G. is hemodynamically stable and, depending on his lab values, he may need the rapid clearance that HD can provide. Mr. G. must be heparinized.

   Peritoneal dialysis—This is a slower procedure and he has a fresh abdominal incision.

   CRRT—Continuous renal replacement therapy

   CAVHD—This removes fluid and waste with minimal heparinization. Removal is gradual, which lessens the risk of hemodynamic changes.

5. Mr. G. is adamantly refusing renal replacement therapy. He refers to his advance directive which lists dialysis as not acceptable. How would you deal with him?

   In order to speak knowledgeably with Mr. G., you should remember that only about 5% of patients with ATN require long-term renal replacement therapy.

CASE STUDY #2

Ms. S., a 45-year-old African American, has been an insulin-dependent diabetic since she was 12. Over the last eight years, she has had deteriorating renal function. She has recently been diagnosed with chronic renal failure and plans have been made for the surgical creation of an arteriovenous (AV) fistula. She is overtly distressed about the process of life-long hemodialysis although she is looking forward to relief from her uremic signs and symptoms, which include pericardial effusion, unrelenting volume overload, renal osteodystrophy, and acidosis. For these reasons, dialysis will be started using a vascular catheter until her fistula matures.

1. What are the psychological ramifications of dialysis?

    Change in body image, (i.e., fistula, equipment)
    Dependency/independence conflicts, (i.e., staff, machine)
    Facing possible death daily

2. What are the goals of hemodialysis?

    Remove excess fluid
    Maintain safe concentration electrolytes
    Establish acid-base balance
    Remove waste products

3. How is the uremic syndrome manifested in the skeletal system?

    Vitamin D becomes Vitamin D_2 in the liver, which becomes Vitamin D_3 (active form) in the kidney
    The body needs Vitamin D_3 to absorb Ca^{++} from the GI tract, which leads to hypocalcemia and hyperphosphatemia, which stimulates parathyroid to produce parathormone and pulls Ca from bones, leading to renal osteodystrophy.

4. Describe the maturation process of an AV fistula.

    It takes approximately six weeks for the vein to become enlarged from arterial pressure of the anastomosed vessel. Once enlarged it is accessible for hemodialysis.

5. What is the pathophysiology of the potential complications of Ms. S.'s pericardial effusion?

    Beck's Triad—increased CVP with JVD, muffled heart sounds, pulsus paradoxus.
    Uremic pericarditis leads to inflammation from circulating waste products, which causes fluid to be secreted to lubricate rub, which leads to pericardial effusion, resulting in pericardial tamponade.

Chapter 12 Case Studies

CASE STUDY #1

Mr. G. is postop abdominal aortic aneurysm (AAA) repair. His hemodynamic status has stabilized but his urine output is low normal at best. Over the next hours, his urine output continues to fall. He develops bilateral crackles, a bounding pulse, and his BP and CVP rise. His BUN, creatinine, and K have also crept higher than his preop values.

1. Explain the reason for Mr. G.'s apparent renal failure.

2. What do you expect to see as Mr. G. moves through the phases of acute tubular necrosis?

3. What is the most sensitive indicator of renal function? Of renal perfusion? Why?

4. Mr. G. needs renal replacement therapy for his fluid over-load, hyperkalemia, and acidotic state. How would you determine which therapy is suitable? Give reasons for each.

5. Mr. G. is adamantly refusing renal replacement therapy. He refers to his advance directive which lists dialysis as not acceptable. How would you deal with him?

Chapter 12 Case Studies

CASE STUDY #2

Ms. S., a 45-year-old African American, has been an insulin-dependent diabetic since she was 12. Over the last eight years, she has had deteriorating renal function. She has recently been diagnosed with chronic renal failure and plans have been made for the surgical creation of an arteriovenous (AV) fistula. She is overtly distressed about the process of life-long hemodialysis although she is looking forward to relief from her uremic signs and symptoms, which include pericardial effusion, unrelenting volume overload, renal osteodystrophy, and acidosis. For these reasons, dialysis will be started using a vascular catheter until her fistula matures.

1. What are the psychological ramifications of dialysis?

2. What are the goals of hemodialysis?

3. How is the uremic syndrome manifested in the skeletal system?

4. Describe the maturation process of an AV fistula.

5. What is the pathophysiology of the potential complications of Ms. S.'s pericardial effusion?

Hypovolemia/Renal Ischemia

or

_____ Sodium Ion Concentration of Blood

↓

_____ production by specialized cells in the juxtaglomerular apparatus (JGA) of kidney

↓

RENIN + ANGIOTENSIN
(produced by the _____)

↓

_____

↓

ANGIOTENSIN I + Converting enzyme in the _____

↓

_____

↙   ↘

Peripheral _____   _____ Release
(from adrenal glands)

↓

_____ and _____ reabsorption and postassium excretion

↓

_____ Circulating volume

↓

_____ BLOOD PRESSURE

DIRECTIONS

Fill in the blanks.

_____

Figure 12–4: Renin-Angiotensin Mechanism

_____ or _____ injury

↓

Tubular wall _____

↙   ↘

_____ Cell swelling   _____ Tubular wall integrity

↓   ↓

_____ of tubular cells   Backleak of _____ into interstitium

↓   ↓

Sloughing of _____ cells (casts)   _____

↓   ↓

_____ of tubules   Retention of nitrogenous wastes (_____)

↓

Impedence to flow of _____

↓

_____

↓

Retention of _____ (Azotemia)

DIRECTIONS

Fill in the blanks.

Figure 12–5: Proposed Mechanisms of Acute Tubular Necrosis Cascade

Symptom	Potential Pathology		
Dysuria	_____		
Dribbling	_____	and	_____
Edema	_____		
Frequency	_____		
Hematuria	_____	and	_____
Hesitancy	_____		
Incontinence	_____	and	_____
Nocturia	_____		
Oliguria	_____	and	_____
Proteinuria	_____		
Pyuria	_____		
Renal colic	_____		
Urgency	_____	and	_____

DIRECTIONS

Fill in the blanks with the potential pathology.

Table 12–6: Renal-Related Symptoms and Their Potential Pathologies

Chapter 13

Hematological and Immune Disorders

TERMINOLOGY

- Adhesion
- Aggregation
- AIDS
- Anemia
- Erythropoietin
- Fibrinogen
- Fibrinolysis
- Hematopoiesis
- Opsonization
- Phagocytosis
- Suppuration
- Thrombocytopenia
- Thrombopoietin

OUTLINE

I. Hematologic anatomy and physiology
  A. Hematopoiesis and hematological function of organs

  B. Characteristics of blood

  C. Components of blood

   1. Plasma

   2. Cells

    a. Erythrocytes: oxygen transport

   1. Reticulocyte

   2. Hematocrit

  b. Leukocytes: immune response

  c. Granulocyte

   1. Neutrophils

    a. Bands

    b. Segmented

---

c. Chemotaxis

d. Phagocytosis

    i. Opsonization

    ii. Suppuration

2. Eosinophil

3. Basophil

d. Nongranular leukocytes

1. Monocytes (macrophages)

2. Lymphocytes: specific immune response

e. Platelets (thrombocytes): blood clotting and hemostasis

1. Hemostasis: prevention of blood loss

2. Coagulation

    a. Intrinsic

    b. Extrinsic

    c. Common

3. Coagulation antagonists and clot lysis

II. Assessment of the hematologic system
  A. Health history

1. Lifestyle factors

2. Physical exam

B. Hematological studies

III. Selected hematological disorders

A. Red blood cell disorders

1. Anemias

a. Pathophysiology

b. Assessment and clinical manifestations

c. Nursing diagnoses

d. Medical interventions

e. Nursing interventions

f. Patient outcomes

B. White blood cell disorders

1. Neutropenia

a. Pathophysiology

b. Assessment and clinical manifestations

c. Nursing diagnosis

d. Medical interventions

e. Nursing interventions

f. Patient outcomes

2. Leukemia

a. Pathophysiology

b. Assessment and clinical manifestations

c. Nursing diagnosis

d. Medical interventions

e. Nursing interventions

C. Bleeding disorders

    1. Disseminated intravascular coagulation (DIC)

        a. Pathophysiology

        b. Clinical manifestations

        c. Nursing diagnosis

        d. Medical interventions

        e. Nursing interventions

        f. Patient outcomes

    2. Thrombocytopenia

        a. Pathophysiology

        b. Assessment and clinical manifestations

        c. Nursing diagnosis

        d. Medical interventions

        e. Nursing interventions

        f. Patient outcomes

        g. White clot syndrome

    3. Other coagulation disorders

        a. Vitamin K deficiency

        b. Liver disease

        c. Massive transfusions, hemophilia, and von Willebrand's

IV. Review of immunological anatomy and physiology

    A. Concepts in immunology

    1. Antigen

        a. Self

        b. Nonself

    2. Tolerance

    3. Specificity

        a. Specific

        b. Nonspecific

B. Organs involved in immunological function

C. Cells involved in immunological function

D. Immune mechanisms

    1. Nonspecific defenses

        a. Epithelial surfaces

        b. Inflammation and phagocytosis

        c. Others

    2. Specific (acquired) defenses

        a. Humoral immunity

            1. Immunoglobulins

        b. Cell-mediated immunity

E. Assessment of immune function

    1. Health history

    2. Dietary practices

    3. Physical

4. Exam

5. Diagnostic tests

F. Selected immunological disorders

   1. Immunocompromise

     a. Primary immunodeficiency

     b. Secondary immunodeficiency

      1. Stress

      2. Age

      3. Malignancy

      4. Chronic disease

      5. Pharmacological agents

6. Therapeutic immunosuppression

7. Infectious diseases

   a. AIDS

     i. Pathophysiology

     ii. Assessment and clinical manifestations

     iii. Nursing diagnoses

     iv. Medical interventions

     v. Research

     vi. Nursing interventions

     vii. Patient outcomes

MULTIPLE CHOICE

1. A process where antigens and damaged cells are removed from tissues is called
   A. opsonization
   B. suppuration
   C. phagocytosis
   D. macrophagia

Correct answer: C

Rationale: This is called phagocytosis.

2. Humoral immunity is mediated by
   A. B lymphocyte
   B. T lymphocytes
   C. B Cells
   D. R Cells

Correct answer: A

Rationale: Humoral immunity is mediated by B lymphocytes; cellular immunity is mediated by B and T lymphocytes and B cells.

3. In a patient with hemostasis accomplished and blood vessel integrity restored, blood flow must be reestablished. This is done through the
   A. humoral system
   B. coagulation pathway
   C. fibrinolytic system
   D. extrinsic pathway

Correct answer: C

Rationale: The enzyme plasmin digests fibrinogen and fibrin. This is called fibrinolysis.

4. Patients with hematologic disorders require a thorough history and physical. What lifestyle factors could alter hematologic functions?

   A. aerobic exercise

   B. anaerobic exercise

   C. substance abuse

   D. working excessively long hours

Correct answer: C

Rationale: Substance abuse, alcohol abuse, occupational exposure to chemicals or radiation, and nutrition can alter hematologic function.

5. Anemia is the reduction the number of circulating RBCs. Identify causes of anemia seen in critical care.

   A. blood loss from trauma or GI bleeding

   B. bone marrow suppression

   C. autoimmune diseases

   D. all of the above

Correct answer: D

Rationale: All of the above can cause anemia.

6. Mr. W. presents with the following signs and symptoms: pallor, fatigue, weakness, and lethargy. He also has periods of tachycardia, palpitation, angina, and systolic murmurs. What is a possible diagnosis?

   A. thrombocytopenia

   B. leukemia

   C. anemia

   D. neutropenia

Correct answer: C

Rationale: Anemia has these general findings.

7. You are caring for a patient in isolation who has the diagnosis of neutropenia. What signs of infections would you expect to see?

   A. increased WBCs

   B. increased phagocyte ability

   C. fever

   D. inflammation, heat, redness, and pain

Correct answer: C

Rationale: Fever may be the only sign of infection that will be present. In neutropenia, there is decreased WBCs, and without phagocytosis typical signs such as inflammation may not appear.

8. Patients with DIC would be expected to have which diagnosis?

   A. fluid volume overload

   B. altered pattern of urinary elimination related to increased renal blood flow

   C. impaired gas exchange related to pulmonary edema

   D. altered tissue perfusion related to abnormal clotting and thrombosis

Correct answer: D

Rationale: Fluid volume is decreased, as is renal blood flow, and pulmonary ischemia such as pulmonary embolism is seen.

9. A controversial treatment of DIC is

   A. blood volume expanders

   B. heparin

   C. transfusions of whole blood

   D. transfusion of packed RBCs

Correct answer: B

Rationale: Heparin is used to prevent further clotting and thrombosis that may lead to organ ischemia, but studies show inconsistent benefits.

10. A nursing measure that should be performed as infrequently as possible in the DIC patient is
    A. accurate measurement of intake and output
    B. lubrication of the skin with frequent turning
    C. taking cuff blood pressures to monitor vital signs
    D. obtaining blood samples through central lines

Correct answer: C

Rationale: Cuff pressures, including noninvasive blood pressure machines, should be used as infrequently as possible.

11. One form of thrombocytopenia is called White Clot Syndrome. This is a complication of what therapy?
    A. blood transfusions
    B. reduced IV fluid administration
    C. heparin administration
    D. dipyridamole administration

Correct answer: C

Rationale: This is a rare complication of heparin therapy, in which white clot aggregates of platelet and fibrin are formed.

12. Immunoglobulins are antibodies produced in specific response to certain antigens. The most common immunoglobulin is unique because it crosses the placenta to provide passive immunity to the newborn. This immunoglobulin is
    A. IgM
    B. IgA
    C. IgG
    D. IgD

Correct answer: C

Rationale: IgG is found in most body fluids.

13. There are currently two tests commonly used for diagnosing HIV. These are
    A. T cell counts for CD4 and CD8
    B. ELISA and Western blot
    C. Total B cell counts and absolute lymphocyte counts
    D. bone marrow aspiration and biopsy

Correct answer: B

Rationale: The diagnostic test for HIV is the ELISA or Western blot. The others assess for cell abnormalities, susceptibility to infection, and white blood cell disorders.

14. Factors of secondary immunodeficiency include
    A. diminished humoral and cell-mediated immunity
    B. deficient production of immunoglobulin
    C. age and stress
    D. acute diseases

Correct answer: C

Rationale: Age, stress, malnutrition, malignancies, and chronic disease cause or are related to secondary immunodeficiency.

15. When is immunosuppression considered therapeutic?
    A. AIDS-related diseases
    B. leukemia
    C. transplantation
    D. malignancies

Correct answer: C

Rationale: Immunosuppression is the ultimate goal in transplantation.

16. AIDS is a disruption of
    A. humoral immunity
    B. cell-mediated immunity
    C. retroviruses
    D. seroconversion

Correct answer: B

Rationale: AIDS is a dysfunction of cell-mediated immunity; HIV causes deficiency in T-helper lymphocytes.

17. What nursing diagnosis would be a top priority in the patient with HIV?

    A. risk for fluid volume deficit

    B. altered nutrition, less than body requirements

    C. risk for injury; seizures related to CNS infection

    D. risk for infection related to disease process

Correct answer: D

Rationale: The top priority is the risk of infection.

18. AIDS research focuses on

    A. antiviral agents

    B. immune modulators

    C. development of a vaccine

    D. all of the above

Correct answer: D

Rationale: The primary goal is development of a vaccine but all are goals of AIDS research.

19. Education of the patients with AIDS and their significant others primarily includes

    A. pain relief and comfort rest measures

    B. diarrhea control through medication

    C. dehydration prevention through adequate intake

    D. understanding of disease transmission and course of disease

Correct answer: D

Rationale: Education regarding disease transmission and the course of the disease decreases isolation and fears and allows for better understanding of treatments and other concerns.

20. Treatment of secondary immunodeficiencies includes

    A. B- and T-cell replacement therapy

    B. bone marrow transplants

    C. somatic gene therapy

    D. antiinfective medications

Correct answer: D

Rationale: All others are treatment measures for primary immunodeficiencies; in secondary immunodeficiencies treatment includes antiinfectives, correction of malnutrition and treatment of underlying conditions.

CASE STUDIES

CASE STUDY #1

Ms. J. is a young married woman admitted to the ICU for symptoms of hepatitis. As you are caring for her you notice oozing around her IV site.

1. What would be a major concern regarding this finding?

   Disseminated intravascular coagulation

2. What do you as the nurse understand about this problem?

   It is always secondary to another disease process. In DIC, procoagulants are released, causing diffuse uncontrolled clotting; large amounts of thrombin are produced so fibrin is deposited in the microvasculature, there is consumption of available clotting factors, and fibrinolysis is stimulated.

3. What clinical manifestations would the nurse look for?

   In subacute DIC only lab reports may reveal the problem. Petechiae, ecchymosis, and purpura can be present on the skin, gingival bleeding and epistaxis may occur and bleeding can be mild to massive. There may be signs of organ ischemia and necrosis resulting from microvasculature clotting (e.g., angina, decreased urine output, GI bleeding, dyspnea, and changes in mental status).

4. Identify primary medical interventions.

   Identifying and treating the underlying cause, stopping abnormal coagulation, and controlling bleeding.

CASE STUDY #2

Mr. H. is admitted to your critical care environment with Kaposi's sarcoma, a malignant tumor of the endothelium. You understand that this is an opportunistic disease related to AIDS.

1. Nursing concerns revolve around what issues?

   Protection of self and others from body fluids, protection of the patient from infectious processes, lack of knowledge and resulting stigma associated with AIDS, terminal illness concerns of patient and family.

2. Rather than focusing on cure, what does care for Mr. H. center on?

   Treatment of opportunistic infections and diseases.

3. Pharmacological researchers are attempting to find a cure for AIDS or at least prolong the lives of AIDS patients. Identify some of the drugs used to tread AIDS.

   Zidovudine, didanosine, zalcitabine, and stavudine.

4. What is the major goal in the United States regarding AIDS?

   Prevention through education, techniques of care of body fluids, and research.

Chapter 13 Case Studies

CASE STUDY #1

Ms. J. is a young married woman admitted to the ICU for symptoms of hepatitis. As you are caring for her you notice oozing around her IV site.

1. What would be a major concern regarding this finding?

2. What do you as the nurse understand about this problem?

3. What clinical manifestations would the nurse look for?

4. Identify primary medical interventions.

CASE STUDY #2

Mr. H. is admitted to your critical care environment with Kaposi's sarcoma, a malignant tumor of the endothelium. You understand that this is an opportunistic disease related to AIDS.

1. Nursing concerns revolve around what issues?

2. Rather than focusing on cure, what does care for Mr. H. center on?

3. Pharmacological researchers are attempting to find a cure for AIDS or at least prolong the lives of AIDS patients. Identify some of the drugs used to tread AIDS.

4. What is the major goal in the United States regarding AIDS?

Exposure to HIV
through sexual contact, contact with infected blood or blood products
(sharing IV drug equipment, transfusions, or accidental exposure), or from
mother to infant during gestation, childbirth, or breast-feeding

↓

HIV Infection
mononucleosis-like illness (in some patients) as HIV infects CD4 cells
and actively replicates—high levels of p24 antigen detectable in serum

↓

Seroconversion
immune system responds—antibodies to HIV produced ELISA and
Western Blot tests positive for HIV antibody

↓

Latency Period
infected individual remains healthy and asymptomatic as many as 12
years, while HIV is slowly replicating in and destroying CD4 cells
CD4+ count > 500/mm^3

↓

**Initial Symptoms of Immunodeficiency and
Declining Immune Function**
lymphadenopathy, night sweats, fever, diarrhea, wasting syndrome,
and neurologic disease; increased susceptibility to herpes viruses,
candidiasis, hairy leukoplakia
CD4+ counts 200–500

↓

Immune System Failure and AIDS
presence of severe opportunistic infections (e.g., PCP, CMV, TB, toxoplas-
mic encephalitis, cryptococcal meningitis) and/or malignancies (e.g.,
Kaposi's sarcoma, primary CNS lymphoma, invasive cervical CA)
CD4+ counts < 200

Figure 13–14. Pathophysiology of HIV infection

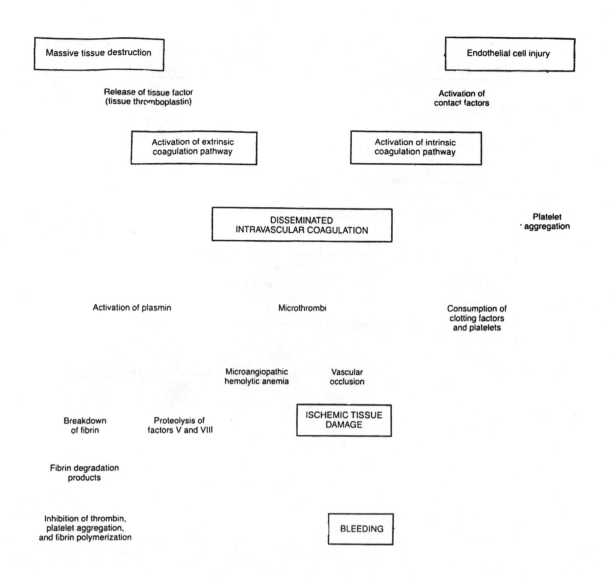

Massive tissue destruction

Release of tissue factor
(tissue thromboplastin)

Endothelial cell injury

Activation of
contact factors

Activation of extrinsic
coagulation pathway

Activation of intrinsic
coagulation pathway

DISSEMINATED
INTRAVASCULAR COAGULATION

Platelet
aggregation

Activation of plasmin

Microthrombi

Consumption of
clotting factors
and platelets

Microangiopathic
hemolytic anemia

Vascular
occlusion

Breakdown
of fibrin

Proteolysis of
factors V and VIII

ISCHEMIC TISSUE
DAMAGE

Fibrin degradation
products

Inhibition of thrombin,
platelet aggregation,
and fibrin polymerization

BLEEDING

DIRECTIONS

Diagram (draw) arrows demonstrating pathophysiology.

Figure 13–8. Pathophysiology of DIC. (From Cotran, R. S., Kumar, V., and Robbins, S. L. (1989): Robbins Pathological Basis of Disease. 4th ed. Philadelphia, W. B. Saunders, Fig. 14–29, p. 700.)

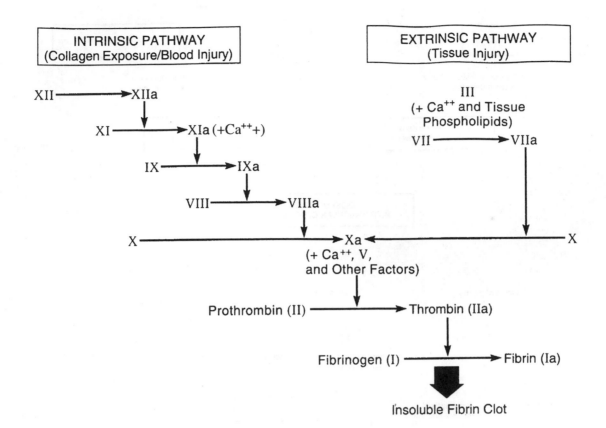

Coagulation pathway study guide.

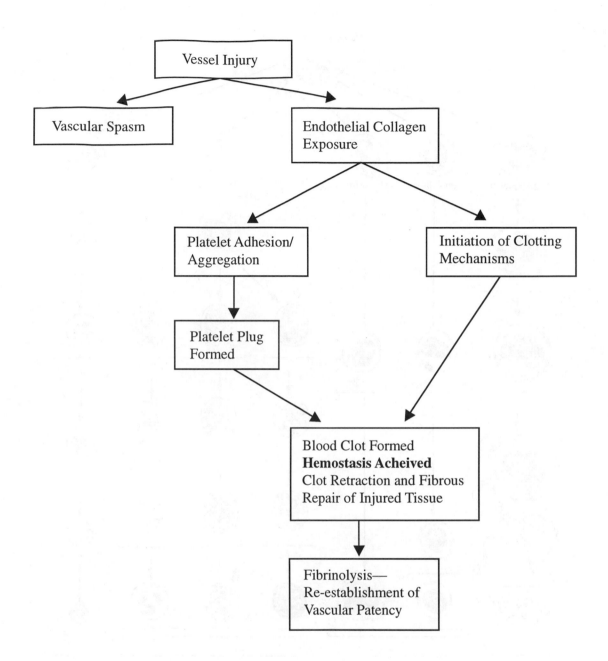

Figure 13–5. Hemostasis study guide.

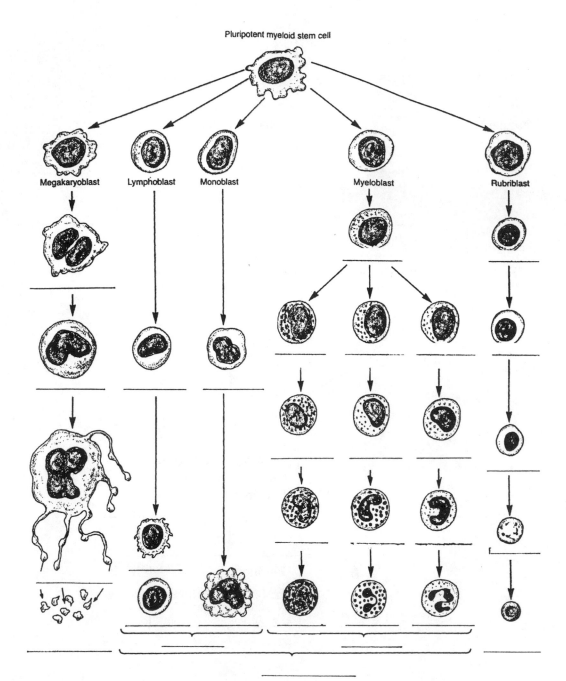

Pluripotent myeloid stem cell

Megakaryoblast   Lymphoblast   Monoblast   Myeloblast   Rubriblast

DIRECTIONS

Fill in the blanks.

Figure 13–1. Origin, development, and structure of thrombocytes, leukocytes, and erythrocytes, from the plurinpotent stem cell. (From Pavel, J., Plunkett, A., and Sink, B., (1993): Basic concepts of hematology. In: J. M. Black and E. Matassarin-Jacobs (eds.). *Luckmann and Sorensen's Medical-Surgical Nursing*. 4th ed. Philadelphia: W. B. Saunders, pp. 1317–1333. Fig 45–2; p. 1320.)

Gastrointestinal Alterations

TERMINOLOGY

- Acini cells
- Anabolism
- Ascites
- Asterixis
- Basal metabolic rate
- Bilirubin
- Catabolism
- Cholecystokinin
- Chvostek's sign (hypocalcemia)
- Chyme
- Conjugated (direct) bilirubin
- Encephalopathy
- Endocrine
- Exocrine
- Gastric lavage
- Gastric mucosal barrier
- Gluconeogenesis
- Glycogenolysis
- Glycogenesis
- Gut
- Haustrations
- Hematemesis
- Hematochezia

- Hepatitis
- Histamine
- Hunger
- Hydrochloric acid
- Intrinsic factor
- Islets of Langerhans
- Intrinsic factor
- Mastication
- Melena
- Pancreas alpha cells
- Pancreas beta cells
- Parasympathetic
- Pepsinogen
- Peristalsis
- Peritoneal lavage
- Pulmonary capillary wedge pressure (PCWP)
- Sclerotherapy
- Splanchnic circulation
- Sympathetic
- Total parenteral nutrition (TPN)
- Trousseau's sign (hypocalcemia)
- Unconjugated (indirect) bilirubin

OUTLINE

I. Introduction: The primary function of the alimentary tract and accessory organs is to provide the body with a continual supply of nutrients; this requires motility, digestion, and absorption. Problems result in disorders: acute GI bleed, acute pancreatitis, and liver failure.

II. Review of anatomy and physiology

   A. GI tract

     1. Gut wall

       a. Mucosa

       b. Gastric mucosal barrier

       c. Submucosa

     2. Oropharyngeal cavity

       a. Mouth

         1. Hunger

         2. Mastication

         3. Salivary glands

           a. Mucous

           b. Amylase

       b. Pharynx

       c. Stomach

         1. Storage of food

         2. Mixing of food (chyme)

         3. Motility

         4. Gastric secretions

           a. Oxyntic gland

             i. Mucous neck cells

             ii. Peptic/chief cells

               a. Hydrochloric acid: normal rate; stimulants (histamine)

               b. Intrinsic factor

               c. Fluid/electrolytes

       d. Small intestine

         1. Structure

           a. Duodenum

             i. Pancreatic juices and bile

             ii. Brunner's glands

           b. Jejunum

           c. Ileum

         2. Movements

         3. Physiology

           a. Digestion

             i. Pancreatic juice enzymes

             ii. Pancreatic juice bicarbonates

           b. Absorption of water, electrolytes, and vitamins

       e. Large intestine

1. Structure

2. Functions

   a. Absorb water and electrolytes

   b. Store fecal material

B. Accessory organs

  1. Pancreas

    a. Structure

    b. Functions: digestion and carbohydrate metabolism

      1. Exocrine: production of digestive enzymes; cells of Acini: inactive form trypsinogen and chymotrypsinogen bicarbonate

      2. Endocrine: produces insulin and glucagon; Islets of Langerhans

  2. Liver

    a. Structure

    b. Function (over 400)

      1. Vascular

        a. Blood storage

        b. Filtration

      2. Secretory

        a. Bile production

        b. Bilirubin metabolism

          i. Unconjugated

          ii. Conjugated

          iii. Jaundice

            a. Hemolytic

            b. Hepatocellular

      3. Metabolic

        a. Carbohydrate

          i. Glycogenesis

          ii. Glycogenolysis

          iii. Gluconeogenesis

        b. Protein

        c. Fat

        d. Production and removal of blood clotting factors

        e. Detoxification

        f. Vitamin and mineral storage

  3. Gallbladder

C. Neural innervation of GI system

D. Hormonal control

E. Blood supply

III. General assessment
  A. History

    1. Past problems

    2. Pain

3. Surgeries

B Inspection

  1. Skin color and texture

  2. Symmetry and contour of abdomen

  3. Masses/pulsation

  4. Peristalsis/movement

C. Auscultation

  1. High-pitched gurgling: air and fluid

  2. Frequency and character: 4–34 per minute

  3. Bruits: vascular

  4. Tympany: gas

  5. Dull: masses

D. Percussion

E. Palpation (performed last)

IV. Nutritional assessment and therapies
  A. Assessment

    1. Basal metabolic rate

    2. Anabolism

    3. Catabolism

    4. Caloric needs

  B. Nutritional therapies

    1. Essential elements

2. Nursing responsibilities

  a. Setup

  b. Fluid and electrolyte balance

  c. Glucose

C. Enteral nutrition

  1. Major types

    a. Intact (complete)

    b. Hydrolyzed (predigested)

  2. Routes

    a. Mouth

    b. Tube

      1. Continuous

      2. Intermittent

  3. Complications

  4. Recommendations to prevent complications

V. Disorders
  A. Acute upper GI bleed

    1. Pathophysiology

      a. Peptic ulcer disease

        1. Duodenal

        2. Gastric

      b. Stress ulcer

    c. Mallory Weiss

    d. Esophageal varices

2. Assessment

    a. Clinical presentation

       1. Hematemesis

       2. Hematochezia

       3. Melena

       4. Other signs

    b. Nursing assessment

       1. Vital signs

       2. Body systems (for shock)

         a. Cool clammy skin

         b. Hyperventilation

         c. BUN

         d. Urine output

         e. Abdominal

       3. History

    c. Medical assessment

       1. Laboratory studies

       2. Barium x-rays and endoscopy

3. Nursing diagnosis

4. Collaborative management

    a. Hemodynamic stabilization

    b. Gastric lavage

    c. Pharmacological therapies

       1. Antacids

       2. Histamine blockers

       3. Mucosal barrier enhancers

       4. Antibiotics

    d. Endoscopic therapies (tamponade vessel)

       1. Sclerotherapy

         a. Morrhuate sodium

         b. Ethanolamine

         c. Tetradecyl sulfate

       2. Thermal

         a. Heater probe

         b. Laser photocoagulation

         c. Electrocoagulation

    e. Surgical therapies

       1. Types

         a. Gastric resections

           i.   Antrectomy

           ii.   Gastrectomy

           iii.   Gastroenterostomy

      iv. Vagotomy

   b. Combined surgeries

      i. Billroth's I

      ii. Billroth's II

   c. Preventing GI complications

      i. Vagotomy

      ii. Pyloroplasty

2. Postoperative care

   a. Fluid and electrolytes

   b. Adequate nutrition

   c. Wound healing

   d. Pain

   e. Lung infections

3. Nursing diagnosis

f. Treatment of variceal bleeds

1. Vasopressin

2. Balloon tamponade

3. Sclerotherapy

4. TIPS procedure

5. Surgical interventions

5. Patient outcomes

a. Fluid volume deficit

b. Anxiety

c. Decreased tissue perfusion

d. Impaired gas exchange

e. Knowledge deficit

f. Fluid volume excess

g. Altered electrolyte balance

h. Encephalopathy

i. Aspiration

j. High risk infection

k. Acute pain

l. Ineffective breathing

B. Acute pancreatitis: mild to hemorrhagic

1. Pathophysiology

   a. Mechanisms unknown

   b. Classified by gradation

      1. Mild: frank pancreatic necrosis absent

      2. Hemorrhagic: leads to high mortality rate

   c. Effects

      1. Hyperglycemia, hypoglycemia, nutritional depletion

      2. Acute: 5 to 7 days then normal

      3. Severe: every organ (fulminating)

4. Local

   a. Inflammation of pancreas

   b. Inflammation of peritoneum and fluid accumulation around peritoneal cavity

5. Multisystem organ dysfunction

   a. DIC

   b. ARDS

   c. Renal failure

   d. Hypocalcemia and hyperlipidemia

   e. Hormone imbalances (e.g., parathyroid)

   f. Pseudocyst

  d. Causes

2. Assessment

  a. History and physical (Table 14–23)

   1. Complaints

    a. Severe abdominal pain

    b. Nausea and vomiting

    c. Fever

    d. Dehydration and hypovolemic shock

  b. Diagnostic tests

   1. Serum amylase and lipase

   2. CT scan and MRI

3. Other common tests

   a. Elevated WBC

   b. Elevated serum glucose

   c. Hypokalemia or hyperkalemia

   d. Hypocalcemia

   e. Decreased serum albumin and protein

  c. Predicting severity (Table 14–25)

3. Nursing diagnosis

4. Nursing and medical interventions

  a. Fluid resuscitation and electrolyte replacement

   1. Fluid replacement

   2. Electrolyte replacement

    a. Calcium

    b. Potassium

    c. Glucose

  b. Supportive therapies

   1. Resting the pancreas

   2. Nutritional support

   3. Comfort

   4. Pharmacological interventions

  c. Treatment of systemic complications

   1. Peritoneal lavage

2. Pulmonary treatments

3. Coagulation abnormalities

4. Cardiovascular monitoring

5. Gastrointestinal

   a. Pseudocyst

   b. Abdominal abscess

   d. Surgical management

5. Patient outcomes

   a. Normal fluid balance

   b. Hemodynamic stability

   c. Diminished pain

   d. Nutritional balance

   e. Gas exchange WNL

   f. Electrolyte balance

   g. Prevent complications

C. Hepatic failure

1. Pathophysiology

   a. Hepatitis

      1. Hepatitis causes

         a. Hepatitis A virus

         b. Hepatitis B virus

         c. Hepatitis C virus

d. Hepatitis D virus

e. Hepatitis E virus

2. Assessment

   a. HAV

      i. Diagnosis

      ii. Signs and symptoms

      iii. Liver function tests

      iv. Communicability, progress, and recovery

   b. HBV

      i. Diagnosis

      ii. Signs and symptoms

      iii. Sequelae

   c. HCV

   d. HDV

   e. HEV

3. Nursing diagnosis

4. Nursing and medical interventions

   a. Rest

   b. Nutritional status (high-carbohydrate, low-protein)

   c. Special precautions

5. Patient outcomes

b. Cirrhosis

   1. Alcoholic

   2. Biliary

   3. Cardiac

   4. Postnecrotic

c. Fatty liver

2. Assessment of hepatic failure

  a. Functional sequelae

    1. Portal hypertension

      a. Hyperdynamic circulation

      b. Esophageal and gastric varices

    2. Reduced liver metabolic processes

      a. Altered carbohydrate metabolism

      b. Altered fat metabolism

      c. Decreased protein metabolism

        i. Ascites

        ii. Bleeding

      d. Loss of Kupffer's cell function

      e. Altered removal of clotting factors

      f. Decreased metabolism and storage

      g. Hormonal imbalances

      h. Impaired drug metabolization

      3. Impaired bile formation and flow

3. Nursing diagnosis

  a. Decreased activity tolerance

  b. Fluid volume deficit

  c. Altered nutrition less than

  d. Risk ineffective breathing

  e. Altered thought processes

  f. Altered renal tissue perfusion

  g. Risk impaired skin integrity

4. Nursing and medical interventions

  a. Diagnostic tests

    1. Lab

    2. Liver biopsy

  b. Supportive therapies

  c. Treatment of complications

    1. Ascites

      a. Nursing assessment and procedures

      b. Medical management

        i. Conservative: bed rest, low sodium diet, fluid restriction, diuretics, monitoring serum and urine

        ii. Paracentesis

        iii. Peritoneovenous shunt

iv. Denver shunt

2. Portal systemic encephalopathy

   a. Causes

   b. Treatment measures

      i. Limit protein intake

      ii. Drugs

         a. Neomycin

b. Lactulose

c. Restrict hepatotoxic drugs

iii. Nursing measures

3. Hepatorenal syndrome (acute renal failure)

5. Patient outcomes

VI. Summary

MULTIPLE CHOICE

---

1. The nurse knows that it is the disruption of the mucosal barrier by certain substances that is believed to play a role in ulcer development. One such substance is
   A. hydrochloric acid
   B. bile salts
   C. tannic acid
   D. nicotine

Correct answer: B

Rationale: The barrier is impermeable to hydrochloric acid; it can be permeable to bile salts, alcohol steroids, and salicylates. Tannic acid and nicotine may increase the production of hydrochloric acid.

2. A sympathetic response could exacerbate a duodenal ulcer due to its inhibitory affect on
   A. parietal cells
   B. Brunner's glands
   C. gastrin
   D. pepsin

Correct answer: B

Rationale: Brunner's glands secrete mucus, which protects the duodenal wall from digestion by gastric juice.

3. One mechanism of the liver that is helpful during episodes of hypoglycemia is
   A. gluconeogenesis
   B. glycogenesis
   C. glycogenolysis
   D. glycogenolyses

Correct answer: C

Rationale: Needed glucose is formed by splitting glycogen stored in the liver; this is termed *glycogenolysis.*

4. Assessment of bowel sounds is done with the diaphragm of the stethoscope; it is important to auscultate for at least five minutes because
   A. bowel sounds are high-pitched, irregular gurgling noises
   B. vascular sounds (bruits) indicate dilated tortuous vessels
   C. Venous hums are heard only in the peritovertebral region
   D. decreased bowel sounds are indicative of acute illness

Correct answer: A

Rationale: Bowel sounds are estimated to occur at from 4–34 per minute and irregularly; therefore, one must listen long enough to determine complete absence.

5. Critically ill patients need nutritional assessment and support early in their illness. The following are included in nutritional assessment. Which is the most common set of parameters utilized by the nurse?
   A. diet history prior to the illness and usual weight
   B. identification of stressors causing increased energy needs
   C. albumin and nitrogen balance
   D. determination of caloric needs using basal energy requirement calculation

Correct answer: C

Rationale: Nitrogen balance indicates whether the body is building or breaking down protein. The normal value of albumin, a protein metabolized by the liver, is 3.5. This maintains blood osmotic pressure and prevents plasma loss from capillaries.

6. Critically ill patients may need nutritional support via total parenteral nutrition (TPN) that is administered by nurses. The nurse does which of the following throughout the therapy?
   A. measures blood sugar via Picca line every six hours
   B. administers insulin daily through Picca line
   C. weighs the patient weekly
   D. maintains sterility of the TPN setup by changing tubing every 24–48 hours

Correct answer: D

Rationale: Prevention of infection of Picca or central line is essential. Measuring of blood sugar is done via finger stick, nothing is administered through the TPN line but TPN, and weights are typically done daily.

7. Patients in intensive care often develop ulcers. The nurse would expect the patient to develop which of the following
   A. duodenal peptic ulcer
   B. gastric peptic ulcer
   C. gastric stress ulcer
   D. Mallory Weiss ulcer

Correct answer: C

Rationale: Stress ulcers are associated with patients who are severely burned, patients with CNS disease, patients who have long term sepsis, and patients who have undergone other events that have adverse effects on gastric mucosa.

8. Mr. W., a 44-year-old businessman, presents with an acute lower gastrointestinal bleed, demonstrating hypotension, tachycardia, and shock. You would also expect to see which of the following?
   A. melena and hematemesis
   B. coffee ground emesis and hematemesis
   C. hematemesis and hematochezia
   D. azotemia and melena

Correct answer: C

Rationale: Hematochezia is demonstrative of a lower acute bleed and massive loss of greater than 1000 ml of blood, and hematemesis is a sign of upper GI bleed. Azotemia is not an expectation and dark stool can occur with both upper and lower GI bleeds.

9. Several pharmacologic therapies are available for the treatment of ulcers. One of these is the use of histamine blockers such as cimetidine or ranitidine. Histamine blockers do which of the following?
   A. act as a direct alkaline buffer
   B. act to block stimulation of parietal cells
   C. act on gastric mucous to reduce the effect of acid secretion
   D. act on bacterium *Helicobacter pylori*

Correct answer: B

Rationale: Histamine blockers block all factors that stimulate parietal cells in the stomach to secrete hydrochloric acid.

10. Treatment of bleeding ulcers can include sclerotherapy and thermal methods of endoscopy. The ultimate purpose of these therapies is to
    A. prevent ARDS as a result of exposure to fatty substances
    B. prevent exsanguination in the case of perforation
    C. tamponade the vessel to stop active bleeding
    D. delay surgery for patients requiring up to eight units of blood

Correct answer: C

Rationale: All endoscopic therapies are performed to tamponade the vessel to stop active bleeding. ARDS is a complication of sclerotherapy, and in the case of a massive bleed surgery is performed to prevent exsanguination; delayed surgery is performed as a result of a patient's needing more than eight units of blood in 24 hours regardless of other treatments.

11. Vasopressin, administered in a dose of 0.2–0.4 U/min. via an infusion, is one treatment for variceal bleeds. Vasopressin acts by
    A. constricting splanchnic blood flow
    B. induce water retention
    C. increasing coronary ischemia
    D. increasing renal flow

Correct answer: A

Rationale: The primary actions of Vasopressin are direct smooth muscle vasoconstriction of GI and lowering portal venous pressure by vasoconstriction.

12. The form of pancreatitis with the highest mortality rate is
    A. acute fatty pancreatitis
    B. acute hemorrhagic pancreatitis
    C. acute cellular pancreatitis
    D. acute trypsin pancreatitis

Correct answer: B

Rationale: Pancreatitis is graded from mild to severe; it is in the severe form that hemorrhage occurs, leading to the highest mortality rate.

13. Death during the first two week of acute pancreatitis is usually a result of
    A. disseminated intravascular coagulation or GI bleeding
    B. ARDS and acute renal failure
    C. hypocalcemia and hyperlipidemia
    D. pancreatic pseudocysts

Correct answer: B

Rationale: The most common complications leading to death in the first two weeks are pulmonary and renal complications.

14. The clinical signs and symptoms of acute pancreatic disease mimic other GI diseases; therefore, lab and diagnostic tests are very important in differential diagnosis. The most specific test is
    A. blood serum triglycerides
    B. serum lipase and amylase
    C. total bilirubin
    D. partial thromboplastin time

Correct answer: B

Rationale: Lipase and amylase are released as the pancreatic cells and ducts are destroyed.

15. Treatment priorities of acute pancreatitis include fluid and electrolyte replacement because hypovolemia and shock are major causes of death early in the disease process. Which of the following therapies would also be appropriate for acute pancreatitis?
    A. avoiding analgesics
    B. nasogastric suction
    C. physical therapy
    D. standard dose insulin therapy

Correct answer: B

Rationale: Nasogastric suction and other therapies to rest the pancreas are a priority, pain control is necessary, rest is more important than physical therapy, and insulin is not always needed and should be given on a sliding scale.

16. A patient diagnosed with acute pancreatitis presenting with persistent abdominal pain, nausea, and vomiting will be ordered a CT scan. What is suspected?
    A. appendicitis
    B. pseudocyst
    C. tumor
    D. gallstones

Correct answer: B

Rationale: Pseudocysts are common complications that present with persistent pain, nausea, and vomiting. A CT is not necessary for gallstones, and appendicitis and tumors are not commonly associated with pancreatitis.

17. Hepatitis is most often caused by
    A. alcoholism
    B. viral disease
    C. AIDS
    D. multisystem organ failure

Correct answer: B

Rationale: The most common cause of hepatitis is viral disease; to date, five have been identified.

18. Maintenance of nutrition is a nursing priority in hepatitis due to the loss of appetite, nausea, and vomiting. What diet is usually recommended?
    A. high-protein, low-carbohydrate
    B. high-fat, low-protein
    C. low-fat, high-protein
    D. low-protein, high-carbohydrate

Correct answer: D

Rationale: A low-protein, high-carbohydrate diet is ordered in small frequent meals with supplements to provide energy and decreased nausea; fats are typically avoided.

19. Important teaching for patients and family members of patients with hepatitis includes
    A. handwashing and personal hygiene techniques
    B. counseling where sexual route transmission is suspected
    C. hepatitis B screening for pregnant women and HIV positive patients
    D. all of the above

Correct answer: D

Rationale: All of these are important to prevent transmission.

20. Patients in hepatic failure may experience gram-negative sepsis. This is a result of damage to which cells?
    A. beta cells
    B. alpha cells
    C. Kupffer's cells
    D. Acini cells

Correct answer: C

Rationale: Kupffer's cells are phagocytic and in hepatic failure their function may be lost, predisposing the patient to severe infections like gram-negative sepsis.

CASE STUDIES

CASE STUDY #1

Ms. J., a 32-year-old woman, is admitted to your unit in negative nitrogen balance. She is ordered enteral feedings because she is comatose from a traumatic head injury. The following questions relate to this patient.

1. The feeding is ordered every four hours. Why are feedings ordered intermittently?

   The stomach normally receives food intermittently.

2. The feeding is delivered via NG tube. Why is it delivered via gravity instead of a more controlled delivery (e.g., via syringe)?

   Use of a syringe increases the risk of pulmonary aspiration.

3. If the feeding tube were placed in the duodenum the feedings would be continuous. Why?

   The duodenum normally receives nutrients in peristaltic waves.

4. Identify complications associated with enteral feedings that the nurse must watch for.

   Tube obstruction, improper placement, diarrhea, dumping syndrome, hyperglycemia, hypercapnia, and electrolyte imbalance.

5. What nursing measures should be carried out to prevent these complications?

   Checking tube placement by utilizing food coloring, checking pH, checking gastric residual, listening for air on syringe injection; using good handwashing technique in preparation of sets and formula, rinsing feeding set with water before adding formulas; monitoring blood sugars, weighing patient daily, checking BUN and electrolytes, using a controller pump to give feedings at constant rate, and flushing feeding tubes before and after administering feedings or medications or every four hours if feeding is continuous.

CASE STUDY #2

Ms. P. has been admitted to your unit with an acute GI bleed as a result of esophageal varices. The first priority for the nurse is to do an assessment of the severity of blood loss, which will include taking vital signs and observing for signs and symptoms of shock.

1. What should the nurse understand about this assessment?

   Vital signs should be taken every 15 minutes; the changes in vital signs relate to the amount of blood lost, the suddenness of blood loss, and the degree of cardiac and vascular compensation. Systolic BP less than 100 mmHg and heart rate greater than 120 per minute reflect loss of 1000 ml or more.

2. The nurse would know that as blood loss exceeds 1000 ml the patient would have cool and clammy skin, would hyperventilate, and would have an increased BUN and decreased urinary output. Why do these changes occur?

   As blood loss increases there is decreased blood to: skin, which becomes cool and clammy; lungs, which causes the patient to hyperventilate to maintain oxygenation; and kidneys, so waste products accumulate in blood and urinary output reflects systemic tissue perfusion.

3. Further assessment findings include hyperactive bowel sounds due to sensitivity of the bowel to blood and either a soft or distended abdomen. The physician orders a CBC, electrolytes, BUN, and arterial blood gases. What would the nurse expect to see in these test results?

   Decreased potassium and sodium due to emesis, increased glucose due to response to stress, increased BUN due to decreased perfusion of kidneys and liver, decreased hematocrit only after extravascular fluid enters vascular space to restore volume (usually after the first few hours).

4. A primary goal is to return Ms. P. to a hemodynamically stable condition. This is done by rapid infusion of fluids through a large-bore intravenous tube. What is the nurse's role in this procedure?

   Gain venous access; administer fluids or blood as ordered; monitor vital signs and signs of hemorrhagic shock; and assess for normal skin color, absence of tachycardia, and adequate urine output.

Chapter 14 Case Studies

CASE STUDY #1

Ms. J., a 32-year-old woman, is admitted to your unit in negative nitrogen balance. She is ordered enteral feedings because she is comatose from a traumatic head injury. The following questions relate to this patient.

1. The feeding is ordered every four hours. Why are feedings ordered intermittently?

2. The feeding is delivered via NG tube. Why is it delivered via gravity instead of a more controlled delivery (e.g., via syringe)?

3. If the feeding tube were placed in the duodenum the feedings would be continuous. Why?

4. Identify complications associated with enteral feedings that the nurse must watch for.

5. What nursing measures should be carried out to prevent these complications?

Chapter 14 Case Studies

CASE STUDY #2

Ms. P. has been admitted to your unit with an acute GI bleed as a result of esophageal varices. The first priority for the nurse is to do an assessment of the severity of blood loss, which will include taking vital signs and observing for signs and symptoms of shock.

1. What should the nurse understand about this assessment?

2. The nurse would know that as blood loss exceeds 1000 ml the patient would have cool and clammy skin, would hyperventilate, and would have an increased BUN and decreased urinary output. Why do these changes occur?

3. Further assessment findings include hyperactive bowel sounds due to sensitivity of the bowel to blood and either a soft or distended abdomen. The physician orders a CBC, electrolytes, BUN, and arterial blood gases. What would the nurse expect to see in these test results?

4. A primary goal is to return Ms. P. to a hemodynamically stable condition. This is done by rapid infusion of fluids through a large-bore intravenous tube. What is the nurse's role in this procedure?

ACUTE PANCREATITIS

Activation of Pancreatic Exocrine Enzymes
(Trypsinogen, Phospholipase A, Elastase)

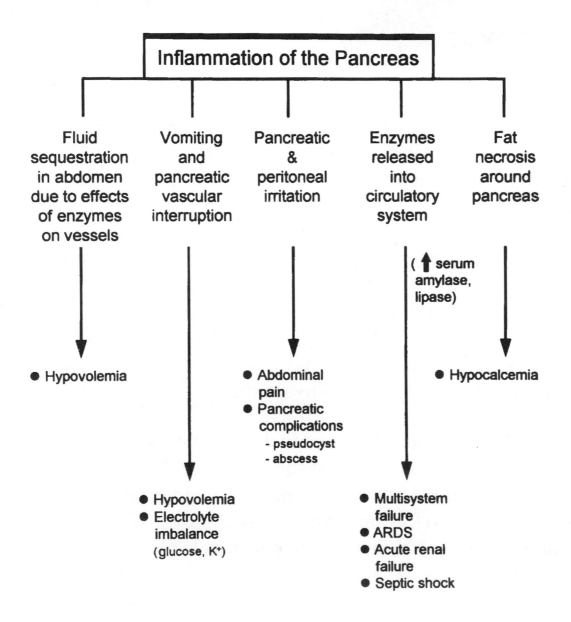

ACUTE PANCREATITIS

Activation of Pancreatic Exocrine Enzymes
(Trypsinogen, Phospholipase A, Elastase)

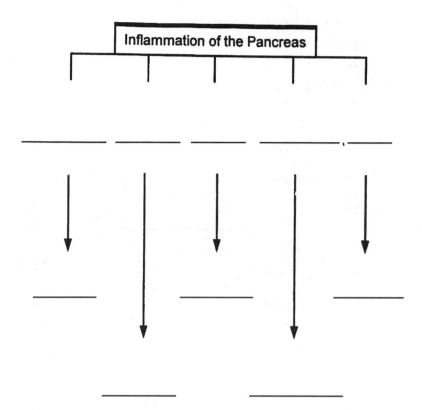

Inflammation of the Pancreas

DIRECTIONS

Fill in the blanks.

ACUTE UPPER GI BLEED

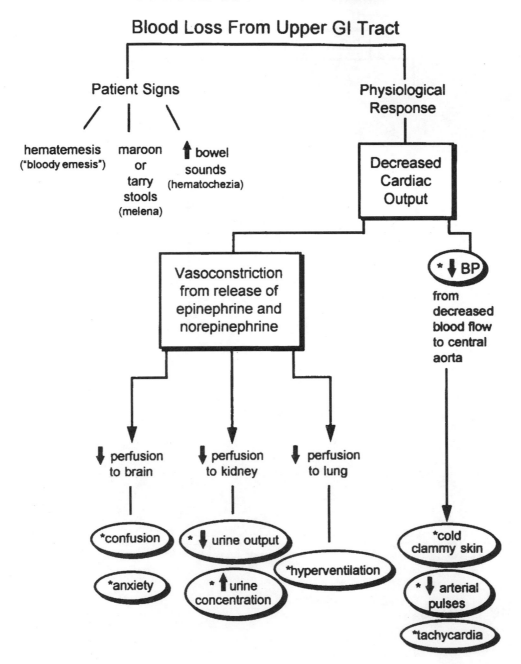

ACUTE UPPER GI BLEED

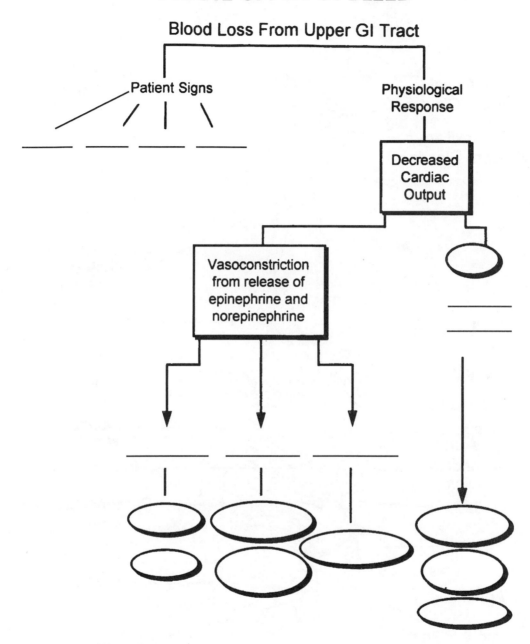

Blood Loss From Upper GI Tract

Patient Signs

_____ _____ _____ _____

Physiological
Response

Decreased
Cardiac
Output

Vasoconstriction
from release of
epinephrine and
norepinephrine

DIRECTIONS

Fill in the blanks.

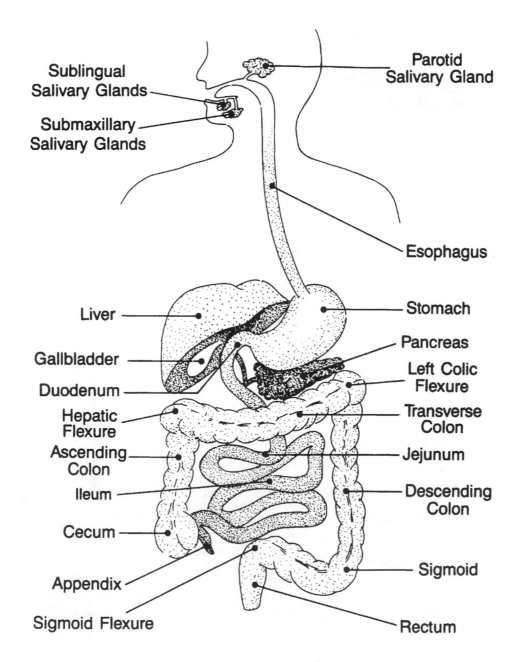

Sublingual Salivary Glands

Submaxillary Salivary Glands

Parotid Salivary Gland

Esophagus

Liver

Stomach

Gallbladder

Pancreas

Duodenum

Left Colic Flexure

Hepatic Flexure

Transverse Colon

Ascending Colon

Jejunum

Ileum

Descending Colon

Cecum

Appendix

Sigmoid

Sigmoid Flexure

Rectum

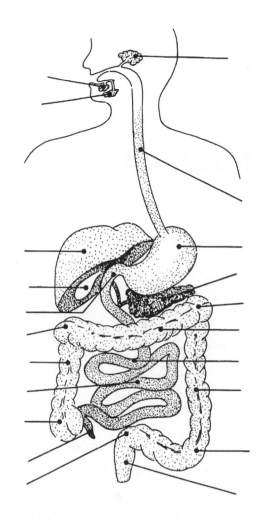

DIRECTIONS

Fill in the blanks.

Chapter

15

Endocrine Alterations

TERMINOLOGY

- Arginine vasopressin
- Diabetes insipidus (DI)
- Diabetic ketoacidosis (DKA)
- Hyperosmolar hyperglycemic nonketotic coma (HHNC)
- Hypoglycemia
- Ketosis

- Kussmaul's respiration
- Lipolysis
- Negative feedback
- Positive feedback
- Syndrome of inappropriate antidiuretic hormone (SIADH)

OUTLINE

I. Introduction

II. Pancreatic endocrine emergencies

    A. Review of physiology

    B. Hyperglycemic crises

        1. Pathophysiology of DKA

        2. Etiology of DKA

        3. Pathophysiology of HHNC

        4. Etiology of HHNC

        5. Assessment

            a. Clinical presentation

            b. Laboratory evaluation

        6. Nursing diagnosis

        7. Nursing and medical intervention

            a. Respiratory support

            b. Fluid replacement

c. Insulin therapy

d. Electrolyte replacement

e. Treatment of acidosis

f. Patient and family teaching

8. Patient outcomes

C. Hypoglycemia

1. Pathophysiology

2. Etiologies

3. Assessment

4. Clinical presentation

5. Laboratory evaluation

6. Nursing diagnosis

7. Nursing and medical interventions

8. Patient outcomes

D. Acute adrenal crisis

1. Review of physiology

2. Pathophysiology

3. Etiology

4. Assessment

   a. Clinical presentation

   b. Neurological system

   c. Cardiovascular system

d. Gastrointestinal system

e. Genitourinary system

f. Integumentary system

g. Laboratory evaluation

5. Nursing diagnosis

6. Nursing and medical interventions

   a. Replacement of fluid and electrolytes

   b. Hormonal replacement

   c. Patient and family education

7. Patient outcomes

E. Thyroid crisis

1. Review of physiology

2. Thyroid storm

   a. Pathophysiology

   b. Etiology

   c. Assessment

      1. Clinical presentation

      2. Neurological disturbances

      3. Cardiovascular disturbances

      4. Integumentary disturbances

      5. Hematopoietic disturbances

      6. Ophthalmic disturbances

7. Laboratory evaluation

d. Nursing diagnosis

e. Nursing and medical interventions

   1. Inhibition of thyroid hormone synthesis

   2. Blockage of thyroid hormone release

   3. Antagonism of peripheral effects of thyroid hormone

   4. Supportive care

   5. Patient education

f. Patient outcomes

3. Myxedema

a. Pathophysiology

b. Etiology

c. Assessment

   1. Clinical presentation

   2. Neurological disturbances

   3. Cardiovascular disturbances

   4. Pulmonary disturbances

   5. Gastrointestinal disturbances

   6. Skeletal disturbances

   7. Integumentary disturbances

   8. Laboratory evaluation

d. Nursing diagnoses

e. Nursing and medical interventions

   1. Thyroid replacement

   2. Restore fluid and electrolyte balance

   2. Supportive care

   3. Patient and family education

f. Patient outcomes

F. Antidiuretic hormone disorders

1. Review of physiology

2. Diabetes insipidus (DI)

   a. Pathophysiology

   b. Assessment

      1. Clinical presentation

      2. Laboratory evaluation

   c. Nursing diagnosis

   d. Nursing and medical interventions

      1. Volume replacement

      2. Hormone replacement

      3. Additional drugs

      4. Nephrogenic DI

      5. Secondary DI

E. Patient and family education

f. Patient outcomes

G. Syndrome of inappropriate antidiuretic hormone (SIADH)

   1. Assessment

      a. Clinical presentation

      b. Central nervous system

      c. Gastrointestinal system

      d. Cardiovascular system

      e. Pulmonary system

f. Laboratory evaluation

   2. Nursing diagnoses

   3. Nursing and medical interventions

      a. Fluid balance

      b. Drug therapy

      c. Nursing

      d. Patient and family education

   4. Patient outcomes

MULTIPLE CHOICE

1. It is important that nurses understand that certain events occur without insulin (e.g., glucose will fail to enter cells and it will accumulate in the blood). What other event would occur?
   A. The insulin will work with growth hormones.
   B. Hypoglycemia results in a decreased level of consciousness.
   C. Cells starve, triggering physiologic process.
   D. Cells starve, triggering thyroid hormones.

Correct answer: C

Rationale: With no insulin, there is *hyper*glycemia, not *hypo*glycemia. Hypoglycemia results in decreased levels of consciousness; insulin works with growth, sex, and thyroid hormones. Lack of insulin results in cells starving but does not trigger thyroid hormones.

2. Diabetic ketoacidosis is
   A. metabolic acidosis
   B. respiratory acidosis
   C. metabolic alkalosis
   D. respiratory alkalosis

Correct answer: A

Rationale: The accumulation of ketoacids from the impairment of metabolism of ketones which result from fatty oxidation is ketoacidosis.

3. Kussmaul's respiration, rapid deep breathing seen in diabetic ketoacidosis (DKA), is the result of the body's need to be rid of
   A. carbonic acid
   B. bicarbonate
   C. H+
   D. lactic acid

Correct answer: A

Rationale: Bicarbonate is decreased in DKA due to osmotic diuresis; therefore, carbonic acid accumulates and the respiratory system attempts to compensate by blowing off carbon dioxide.

4. The fruity breath of a patient with DKA is the result of
   A. ketones
   B. H+
   C. acetone
   D. lactic acid

Correct answer: C

Rationale: As the patient becomes more acidic he or she is less able to metabolize the ketones that form acetone, which gives the fruity breath.

5. Patients with hyperosmolar hyperglycemic nonketotic coma (HHNC) have a higher mortality rate than patients with diabetic ketoacidosis. This is due in part to the fact that these patients are older and commonly have other medical problems. What is the major reason for this high mortality rate?
   A. DKA happens rapidly
   B. HHNC happens insidiously
   C. HHNC causes cellular dehydration
   D. DKA causes cellular dehydration

Correct answer: B

Rationale: By the time patients with HHNC seek medical attention they are profoundly dehydrated and hyperosmolar; DKA happens more rapidly.

6. What is one sign nurses must be especially aware of when diagnosing elderly patients with DKA or HHNC?
   A. polydipsia
   B. polyphagia
   C. polyuria
   D. polylypomia

Correct answer: A

Rationale: The elderly have a decreased sense of thirst so polydipsia may be missing in this group of patients.

7. Patients with HHNC who develop pneumonia may have clear auscultation. What causes this?
   A. the pathophysiology of acidosis
   B. intravascular dehydration
   C. intracellular hydration
   D. hyperosmolarity

Correct answer: B

Rationale: As both intracellular and intravascular volume are depleted vomiting becomes a problem with worsened dehydration, decreased urine output, and even clear lungs in the presence of pneumonia.

8. In HHNC the laboratory results are similar to DKA with three major exceptions. What differences would you expect to see in HHNC?
   A. higher serum glucose, higher osmolality, and greater ketosis
   B. higher serum glucose, higher osmolality, and milder ketosis
   C. lower serum glucose, lower osmolality, and greater ketosis
   D. lower serum glucose, lower osmolality, and milder ketosis

Correct answer: B

Rationale: In HHNC there is no or milder ketosis and higher glucose and osmolality.

9. Nursing responsibilities are multiple in DKA and HHNC. What is the first priority in managing these life-threatening disorders?
   A. fluid replacement to prevent shock
   B. insulin therapy
   C. assessment of airway, breathing, and circulation
   D. electrolyte replacement, especially for potassium

Correct answer: C

Rationale: The first priority is assessment and then support of airway, breathing, and circulation (e.g., oral airways, oxygen therapy, elevating the head of bed, and sometimes intubation).

10. When a patient experiences hypoglycemia the presenting signs related to lack of glucose to the brain include headache, irritability, mental status changes, dizziness, and paresthesias. Signs related to activation of the sympathetic nervous system are
    A. bradycardia, diaphoresis, pallor, cool clammy skin
    B. tachycardia, diaphoresis, pallor, warm clammy skin
    C. tachycardia, diaphoresis, pallor, cool clammy skin
    D. bradycardia, diaphoresis, flushed warm clammy skin

Correct answer: C

Rationale: Epinephrine release causes cool clammy skin, pallor, tremors, palpitations, and tachydysrhythmias.

11. Cortisol is released in response to
    A. renin-angiotensin system
    B. increased of blood glucose
    C. anterior pituitary release of ACTH
    D. decreased plasma sodium

Correct answer: C

Rationale: Cortisol is released in response to ACTH release from the anterior pituitary, which is part of a negative feedback system.

12. Deficiency of aldosterone results in decreased sodium and water retention, decreased circulating volume, and increased potassium and hydrogen ion reabsorption. This happens only in primary adrenal insufficiency; why does this not occur in secondary adrenal insufficiency?
    A. at least 90% of the adrenals must be destroyed before these symptoms show themselves
    B. aldosterone secretion is not dependent on ACTH
    C. ACTH deficiency does not cause this type of deficiency
    D. aldosterone secretion is dependent on ACTH

Correct answer: B

Rationale: Secondary adrenal insufficiency is a result of interference with ACTH secretion or suppression of normal secretion of corticosteroids, which results in deficiencies of glucocorticoids, not mineralocorticoids.

13. Patients with HIV are a new group at risk for adrenal insufficiency. This is because
    A. cytomegalovirus infection destroys over 90% of the adrenals
    B. HIV patients receive trimethoprim and ketoconazole
    C. HIV patients receive large doses of corticosteroids
    D. cytomegalovirus infection destroys less than 90% of the adrenals

Correct answer: B

Rationale: Although the adrenal gland is a site of cytomegalovirus infection, it is rare that it destroys over 90% of the gland. However, these patients are treated with trimethoprim and ketoconazole, which are also known to suppress adrenal function.

14. Hyperthyroidism should be suspected in which of the following?

    A. a patient who demonstrates unusual brady-cardia while asleep

    B. a patient who demonstrates tachycardia while asleep

    C. a patient who demonstrates unregulated hypometabolism

    D. a patient whose fibrillation responds to digoxin

Correct answer: B

Rationale: Patients who have sinus tachycardia or whose atrial fibrillation does not slow in response to digoxin should be suspected to have hyperthyroidism.

15. The severity of a thyroid storm can be determined by

    A. levels of TSH

    B. levels of thyroxine

    C. organ responsiveness to thyroid hormone

    D. degree of thyroid organ destruction

Correct answer: C

Rationale: The severity of the hyperthyroid state is not necessarily indicated by the serum levels of thyroid hormone but more by tissue and organ responsiveness to the hormone.

16. Iodide agents can be given to inhibit the release of thyroid hormone. Possible side effects of iodide agents include metallic taste, inflammation of the salivary glands, tinnitus, headaches, diarrhea, and gastritis. One such iodide medication is

    A. Oragrafin

    B. lithium carbonate

    C. Lugol's solution

    D. Iopanoate

Correct answer: B

Rationale: Lugol's solution or potassium iodide is usually given 1–2 hours after antithyroid drugs to prevent the iodide from being used to synthesize more thyroxine.

17. A patient admitted in a coma with a surgical scar on the lower neck or who has a history of unusual sensitivity to medications or narcotics would be suspected to have what?

    A. hyperthyroidism

    B. thyroid storm

    C. myxedema

    D. Lugol's reaction

Correct answer: C

Rationale: Myxedema coma due to hypothyroidism takes many months to develop and should be suspected in patients who have known thyroid history, lower neck surgical scar, or are unusually sensitive to narcotics.

18. Neurogenic diabetes insipidus is primarily controlled with the administration of exogenous ADH preparations. These drugs

    A. correct hypernatremia and replace free water

    B. replace ADH and enable kidneys to conserve water

    C. enhance water reabsorption

    D. restrict sodium depletion

Correct answer: B

Rationale: The exogenous ADH, usually Desmopressin, a synthetic analog of vasopressin, replaces or supplements depleted ADH to enable the kidneys to conserve water.

19. In laboratory evaluations, the hallmark of SIADH is

    A. hypernatremia and hyperosmolality

    B. hyponatremia and hypoosmolality

    C. hyperkalemia and hyperosmolality

    D. hypokalemia and hypoosmolality

Correct answer: B

Rationale: The hallmark of SIADH is hyponatremia and hypoosmolality in the presence of inappropriately concentrated urine. Hyponatremia and hypoosmolality result from water retention.

20. Clinical research in nursing is essential to the improvement of care to critically ill patients. Results of a study on fingerstick glucose analysis of patients in shock revealed

   A. fingerstick measurement is better for these patients

   B. fingerstick measurement is the same as venous draw

   C. fingerstick measurement should not be used

   D. no significant findings could be established

Correct answer: C

Rationale: The findings revealed that fingerstick blood samples should not be used for bedside glucose analysis in patients who may have inadequate tissue perfusion.

CASE STUDIES

CASE STUDY #1

Mr. Y. had Addison's disease a result of primary mechanisms leading to hypofunction of the adrenal gland. He was just at a business meeting where everything seemed to fall apart and he talks about "this being the straw that broke the camel's back." You know that patients with chronic hypofunction of the adrenal gland are at special risk during crisis.

1. What would you look for in Mr. Y.'s clinical presentation at this time?

Clinical presentations relate to history of drugs such as steroids, phenytoin, barbiturates, and rifampicin. The nurse should ask questions about illness (e.g., infection, cancer, autoimmune disease, diseases treated with steroids, radiation to head or abdomen, or HIV). Look for a family history or previous diagnosis history of autoimmune disease or Addison's disease. Patient may report weight loss or appetite loss, and fatigue, dizziness, weakness, darkening of skin, low blood glucose unresponsive to therapy, salt craving; he may also complain of headache, confusion, listlessness, hypotension, tachycardia, cold pale skin, and decreased urine output.

2. Laboratory tests done on Mr. Y. include plasma cortisol levels. Discuss what you understand about this lab work.

You should expect a decreased plasma cortisol but this will not indicate whether this is a primary or secondary adrenal insufficiency. You can expect a plasma cortisol less than 10 mg/dl in severe adrenal insufficiency. If the patient is stressed and has a "normal" plasma cortisol, consider adrenal insufficiency. The ACTH level will vary depending on the primary or secondary cause of adrenal insufficiency.

CASE STUDY #2

A 44-year-old woman is admitted to the ICU with complications of her long-term insulin-dependent diabetes—adult onset. You understand that there are many signs and symptoms of DKA and HHNK, so you need to do an assessment of this patient.

1. What are the nursing diagnoses you may develop for the patient who may have DKA or HHNK?

   Fluid volume deficit related to hyperglycemia and osmotic diuresis, effects of vomiting.

   Ineffective breathing pattern and/or impaired gas exchange related to Kussmaul's respiration to compensate for acidosis (DKA); effects of level of consciousness on respiratory status.

   Sensory/perceptual alterations related to metabolic electrolyte abnormalities.

   Electrolyte imbalance related to hyperglycemia, osmotic diuresis, vomiting, acidosis, and treatment regimen.

   Acid-base imbalance: acidosis (DKA) related to ketone and hydrogen ion accumulation, hypoperfusion from dehydration, and decreased bicarbonate reserve.

   Knowledge deficit related to disease process, monitoring, and treatment regimen.

2. What are the primary objectives for the patient with DKA or HHNK and what interventions will be implemented?

   The primary objectives are respiratory support, fluid and electrolyte replacement, administration of insulin to correct hyperglycemia, correction of acidosis in DKA, prevention of complications, and patient teaching and support.

   Treatments include assessment of the above, airway and breathing support through use of oral airways and oxygen therapy, establishment of intravenous access and rehydration, monitoring for signs of hypovolemic shock, administering normal saline (0.9%) for replacement of extracellular fluid volume deficits (usually at rapid rates initially), replacement of insulin for normal uptake of glucose by cells, monitoring serum glucose levels every 1–2 hours while on continuous insulin drip therapy, electrolyte replacement, and treatment of acidosis when required by intravenous bicarbonate to bring pH up to 7.10.

Chapter 15 Case Studies

CASE STUDY #1

Mr. Y. had Addison's disease a result of primary mechanisms leading to hypofunction of the adrenal gland. He was just at a business meeting where everything seemed to fall apart and he talks about "this being the straw that broke the camel's back." You know that patients with chronic hypofunction of the adrenal gland are at special risk during crisis.

1. What would you look for in Mr. Y.'s clinical presentation at this time?

2. Laboratory tests done on Mr. Y. include plasma cortisol levels. Discuss what you understand about this lab work.

CASE STUDY #2

A 44-year-old woman is admitted to the ICU with complications of her long-term insulin-dependent diabetes—adult onset. You understand that there are many signs and symptoms of DKA and HHNK, so you need to do an assessment of this patient.

1. What are the nursing diagnoses you may develop for the patient who may have DKA or HHNK?

2. What are the primary objectives for the patient with DKA or HHNK and what interventions will be implemented?

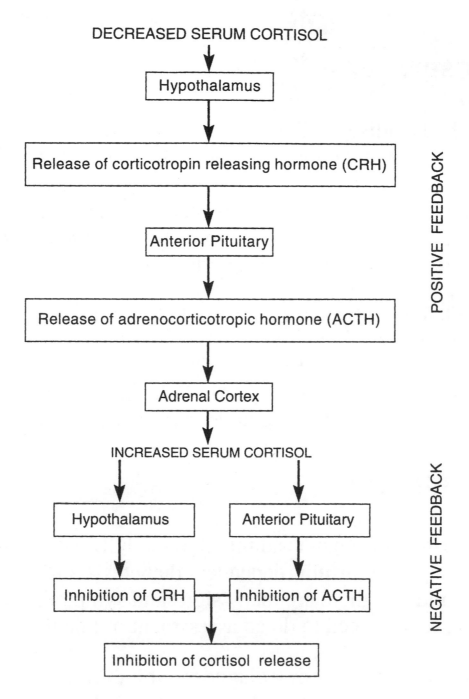

DECREASED SERUM CORTISOL

Hypothalamus

Release of corticotropin releasing hormone (CRH)

Anterior Pituitary

Release of adrenocorticotropic hormone (ACTH)

Adrenal Cortex

INCREASED SERUM CORTISOL

Hypothalamus　　Anterior Pituitary

Inhibition of CRH　　Inhibition of ACTH

Inhibition of cortisol release

POSITIVE FEEDBACK

NEGATIVE FEEDBACK

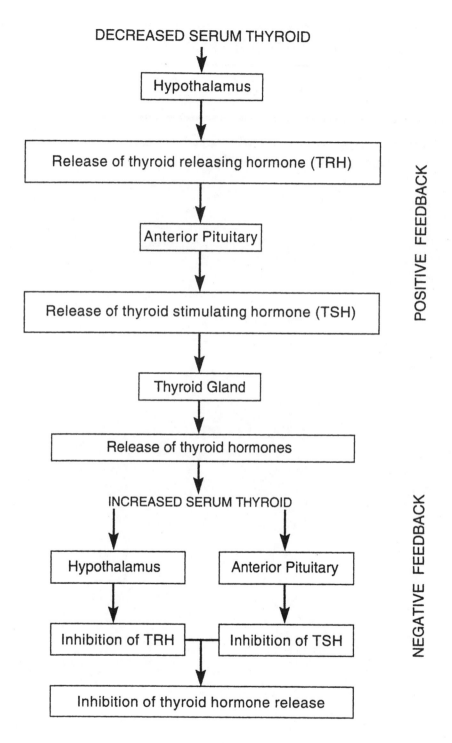

Table 15–2. CALCULATION FOR ANION GAP

$$Na^+ - (Cl^- + HCO_3^-)$$

Normal value 12–14 mEq/L; elevated value indicates accumulation of acids associated with DKA.

Table 15–5. MANIFESTATIONS OF DIABETIC KETOACIDOSIS AND HYPEROSMOLAR HYPERGLYCEMIC NONKETOTIC COMA

	DKA	HHNC
Pathophysiology	Insulin deficiency resulting in cellular dehydration and volume depletion, acidosis, and protein catabolism	Insulin deficiency resulting in dehydration, hyperosmolality, and impaired renal function
Health history	History of Type I DM (use of insulin) Signs and symptoms of hyperglycemia prior to admission Can also occur in Type II DM in severe stress	History of Type II DM (non–insulin-dependent) Signs and symptoms of hyperglycemia prior to admission Occurs most frequently in elderly, with preexisting renal and cardiovascular disease
Onset	Develops quickly	Develops insidiously
Clinical presentation	Flushed, dry skin Dry mucous membranes Decreased skin turgor Tachycardia Hypotension Kussmaul's respirations Acetone breath Altered level of consciousness Polydipsia Polyuria Nausea and vomiting Anorexia	Flushed, dry skin Dry mucous membranes Decreased skin turgor (may not be present in elderly) Tachycardia Hypotension Shallow respirations Altered level of consciousness (generally more profound and may include absent deep tendon reflexes, paresis, and positive Babinski's sign)
Diagnostics	Elevated plasma (average: 675 mg/dl) and urine glucose levels Arterial pH <7.30 Decreased bicarbonate Positive serum and urine ketoacids Azotemia Electrolytes vary with state of hydration; often hyperkalemic on presentation despite marked body deficit Plasma hyperosmolality increased due to hemoconcentration	Elevated plasma glucose (usually <1000 mg/dl) Arterial pH <7.30 Bicarbonate >15 mEq/L Absence of significant ketosis Azotemia Electrolytes vary with state of hydration; often hypernatremic, which contributes to hyperosmolality Plasma hyperosmolality (>330 mOsm/kg)

Table 15-8. CAUSES OF HYPOGLYCEMIA

Excess Insulin/Oral Hypoglycemics
Insulin
Oral hypoglycemics
Islet cell tumors (insulinomas)
Liver disease (impaired metabolism of insulin)
Renal disease (impaired inactivation of insulin)
Autoimmune phenomenon
Drugs that potentiate action of antidiabetic
    medications (propranolol, oxytetracycline)
Elderly patients on sulfonylureas

Underproduction of Glucose

Heavy alcohol
Poor nutrition
Drugs: aspirin, disopyramidine (Norpace), haloperidol
    (Haldol)
Underproduction by liver
Hormonal causes

Too Rapid Utilization of Glucose

GI surgery
Extrapancreatic tumor
Strenuous exercise

Table 15–9. SIGNS AND SYMPTOMS OF HYPOGLYCEMIA

Decrease in Blood Sugar

Rapid	Prolonged
Activation of sympathetic nervous system	Inadequate glucose supply to neural tissues
Epinephrine release from adrenal medulla	Neuroglycopenia
Nervousness	Headache
Apprehension	Restlessness
Tachycardia	Difficulty speaking
Palpitations	Difficulty thinking
Pallor	Visual disturbances
Diaphoresis	Altered consciousness
Dilated pupils	Coma
Tremulousness	Convulsions
Fatigue	Change in personality
General weakness	Psychiatric reactions
Headache	Maniacal behavior
Hunger	Catatonia
	Acute paranoia

Chapter 16

Burns

TERMINOLOGY

- Deep partial thickness injury
- Superficial partial thickness injury
- Full thickness injury

OUTLINE

I.   Introduction
   A. Phases of dysfunction

   B. Three treatment phases

II. Anatomy and physiology of the skin
   A. Layers of skin

      1. Epidermis

      2. Dermis

   B. Depth of injury

      1. Partial thickness

      2. Full thickness

      3. Three zones of thermal injury

III. Pathophysiology
   A. Local response

   B. Systemic response

      1. Hypofunction

      2. Hyperfunction

   C. Host defense mechanisms

   D. Pulmonary response

   E. Renal response

   F. Gastrointestinal response

   G. Metabolic response

IV. Types of burn injuries
   A. Thermal injuries

   B. Chemical injuries

   D. Electrical injury

   E. Nonburn injury

      1. Toxic epidermal necrolysis

2. Staphylococcal scalded skin

V. Assessment
   A. Resuscitative phase

   1. Respiratory

   2. Cardiovascular

   3. Neurological

   4. Blood, fluid, and electrolytes

   5. Renal

   6. Gastrointestinal

   7. Integumentary

   8. Psychosocial

   B. Acute phase

   1. Respiratory

   2. Cardiovascular

   3. Neurological

   4. Blood, fluid, and electrolytes

   5. Renal

   6. Gastrointestinal

   7. Integumentary

   8. Psychosocial

VI. Nursing diagnoses
    A. Resuscitative phase

    B. Acute phase

VII. Collaborative interventions
    A. Findings at the scene

    B. Accurate history of events leading to burn injury

    C. Preparation for transport

    D. Emergency department intervention—resuscitative phase

    1. Treatment specific to type

    2. Preparation for transfer to burn center

       a. Assessment

       b. Planning

       c. Nursing guidelines

          1.

          2.

          3.

          4.

          5.

          6.

          7.

          8.

    E. Acute care interventions—critical care burn unit

    1. Specific treatments for types of injuries

    2. Pain control in resuscitative and acute care phases

    3. Infection control

4. Wound management

    a. Types of treatment

        1. Open

        2. Occlusive

    b. Autograft treatment

5. Special areas of concern

    a. Facial burns

    b. Ear burns

    c. Eye burns

    d. Hands and feet

6. Nutritional considerations

7. Psychosocial considerations

F. Discharge planning

VIII. Patient outcomes

    A. Pulmonary

    B. Fluid and electrolytes

    C. Cardiovascular

    D. Pain

    E. Infection and normothermia

    F. Tissue integrity

    G. Gastrointestinal and stress response

    H. Nutrition

    I. Physical mobility

    J. Patient and family coping

IX. Summary

MULTIPLE CHOICE

1. You are caring for a patient with an electrical burn injury. One major complication of electrical injury is acute renal failure. What causes this?
   A. inadequate fluid resuscitation
   B. muscle destruction
   C. direct effect of current
   D. hemochromogen in small volume of urine

Correct answer: D

Rationale: Hemochromogen in small volume of urine results in renal failure.

2. What are the clinical indicators that your patient has respiratory injury related to burns?
   A. signs of hypoxemia
   B. presence of soot around mouth and nose
   C. abnormal breath sounds
   D. all of the above

Correct answer: D

Rationale: All of the above are signs of respiratory injury related burns, in addition to respiratory difficulty and abnormal blood gas values.

3. Fluid resuscitation consensus formula is 2–24 ml/L × weight (Kg) × percentage of burn. How is the total fluid requirement divided for treatment?

   A. first eight hours: ¼ total fluids
   B. first eight hours: ⅛ total fluids
   C. first eight hours: ½ total fluids
   D. individually calculated

Correct answer: C

Rationale: The administration rate is ½ in the first eight hours, ¼ in the second eight hours, and ¼ in the third eight hours.

4. There are guidelines for burn center referral. What percentage of the total body surface area of full thickness injury should result in transfer?

   A. 5%
   B. 10%
   C. 15%
   D. 20%

Correct answer: A

Rationale: If even only 5% of full thickness burns exist the patient should be transferred; other criteria related to types of burns and partial thickness or full thickness injuries (see Table 16–6).

5. One drug utilized in treating burns is silver nitrate. It is used because it

   A. is effective against most gram-positive and gram-negative wound pathogens
   B. is effective against wide spectrum wound pathogens and fungal infections
   C. functions as a dermal layer to the skin
   D. is used as a temporary wound cover

Correct answer: B

Rationale: Silver nitrate is effective against wide spectrum wound pathogens and fungal infections.

6. There are three phases of treatment in burn care. The most crucial phase is the

   A. acute phase
   B. resuscitative phase
   C. rehabilitative phase
   D. dysfunctional phase

Correct answer: B

Rationale: The resuscitative phase lasts for 48 hours and is the most crucial period for the patient.

7. Deep partial thickness injuries can heal spontaneously but they are most often

   A. covered with biocclusive dressings
   B. debrided
   C. excised and grafted
   D. treated with hyperbaric therapy

Correct answer: C

Rationale: These injuries will achieve better functional and cosmetic results if excised and grafted.

8. There are complex interactions that lead to host defense mechanisms. These result in

   A. overstimulation of suppressor T cells
   B. complement activation
   C. depression of T-helper and T-killer cell activity
   D. all of the above

Correct answer: D

Rationale: The mechanism for many immune defects that occur with extensive burn injury is unclear but the end result is all of the above.

9. Full thickness burn injury can occur in 3–5 seconds at what temperature?

   A. 44° C
   B. 60° C
   C. 70° C
   D. 80° C

Correct answer: B

Rationale: It takes only 60° C, or 140° Fahrenheit, to cause a burn; this is the temperature most hot water heaters are set at.

10. Electrical injury results in tissue damage as electrical energy is converted to heat. The least resistive tissue to electrical injury is
    A. bone
    B. muscle
    C. fat
    D. nerve

Correct answer: D

Rationale: Nerve tissue is least resistive to electrical energy.

11. Types of donor site dressings include fine mesh gauze, zeroform, opsite, duoderm, and vigilon. Which of the following best describes vigilon?
    A. translucent, nonabsorbent, with no reactive surface material
    B. colloidal suspension on a polyethylene mesh
    C. cotton gauze
    D. mesh that contains 3% bismuth tribromophenate in petrolatum

Correct answer: B

Rationale: Vigilon is a colloidal suspension that provides a moist environment and is permeable to gases and water vapor.

12. What zone of thermal injury is the site of minimal cell involvement?
    A. coagulation
    B. hyperemia
    C. stasis
    D. hyperstasis

Correct answer: B

Rationale: Coagulation is the site of irreversible skin death; hyperemia is the site of minimal cell involvement; stasis is potentially salvageable from cell death.

13. The rule of nines is used as an assessment tool. What variation is taken into consideration in adjusting this rule for children?
    A. extremity size
    B. proportion of head size
    C. proportion of back size
    D. there is no variation

Correct answer: B

Rationale: A child's head is proportionately larger related to lower extremities.

14. The first priority in prehospital interventions is to stop the burning. The nurse knows that one specific difference in the care of a person who has a chemical burn rather than a thermal burn is
    A. cooling of the area
    B. removal of the clothing
    C. removal of tar at the scene
    D. remove from the source of burning

Correct answer: B

Rationale: Clothing should be removed with the chemical burn injury because the chemicals will continue to damage the patient if left intact. Clothing is left on in thermal injuries.

15. Ice is an important treatment at the emergency scene.
    A. true
    B. false

Correct answer: B

Rationale: False, because heat loss occurs very rapidly in major burn injury.

16. Large-bore IVs are started in an unburned peripheral area of the body. Which of the following is incorrect?
    A. Catheters are places distal to circumferential burns.
    B. Central lines should not be used.
    C. Ringer's lactate is infused at 500 ml/hour initially.
    D. The needle size should be #16 or #18.

Correct answer: A

Rationale: Catheters should not be placed distal to circumferential burns.

17. The nurse can expect that patients with electrical burns or crush injuries will require _____ volumes of resuscitative fluids.
    A. lesser
    B. greater
    C. equivalent

Correct answer: B

Rationale: Greater volume of fluids is required due to the hemochromogens released as a result of severe deep tissue damage not always apparent.

18. Nurses need to assess burn patients before transport to minimize complications. The first priority is
    A. thermoregulation
    B. mechanisms to prevent aspiration
    C. adequate circulatory support
    D. a secure patent airway

Correct answer: D

Rationale: A patent airway remains a top priority in all critically ill patients.

19. When patients arrive at the burn unit critical indices are again assessed. The frequency of assessment should be
    A. q15m
    B. q1h
    C. q2hr
    D. q shift

Correct answer: B

Rationale: The assessments should be done at least hourly.

20. Pain management for burn patients can be achieved by administering
    A. morphine 3–5 mg
    B. meperidine 100–200 mg
    C. Tylenol with 60 mg codeine
    D. Advil 650 mg

Correct answer: A

Rationale: Morphine at 3–5 mg, preferably IV, is effective for pain management.

CASE STUDIES

CASE STUDY #1

Mr. C. has been a firefighter for 15 years and is very experienced in safety. However, today's fire took the lives of several firefighters and resulted in Mr. C.'s being burned over 30% of his body.

1. What should nursing care of Mr. C. during the acute phase include?

   Assess respiratory rate and character q1h, breath sounds q4h and level of consciousness q1h, monitor oxygen saturation q1h, obtain and evaluate ABGs as needed, administer humidified oxygen as ordered, cough and deep breathe q1h while awake, and suction q1–2 h as needed, elevate head of bed to facilitate lung expansion, and schedule activities to avoid fatigue.

2. Mr. C. is going to be transferred to a burn unit. What is a major concern for the nurse?

   Safety

3. It is expected that Mr. C. will need an autograft for his facial burns. What assessments and interventions are expected of the nurse for a patient receiving an autograft?

   Assess integument twice daily, pad pressure areas, assess need for special beds, remove BP cuff from areas of burned skin after each reading, check circulation distal to restraints q1h, check circulation in digits, immobilize skin graft sites for 5–7 days postgrafting to promote graft adherence, and moisten meshed graft dressings or roll sheet grafts as ordered to promote skin graft adherence.

CASE STUDY #2

Mr. G. was golfing during a storm. He attempted to leave the golf course as it started to rain but was struck by lighting as he approached a tree. Mr. G. has a wife and three children.

1. What are some assessments and interventions for the patient and family dealing with this life-threatening crisis?

   Support adaptive coping mechanisms, use interventions to reduce patient fatigue and pain, promote use of group support sessions for patients and families, orient patient and family to unit and support services, reinforce information frequently, involve patient and family in treatment goals and plan of care.

2. If these interventions are successful what outcomes should the nurse expect?

   Patient and/or family verbalizes goals of treatment regimen, demonstrates knowledge of support systems that are available, are able to express concerns and fears, coping is functional and realistic for phase of hospitalization; family processes are at precrisis level.

Chapter 16 Case Studies

CASE STUDY #1

Mr. C. has been a firefighter for 15 years and is very experienced in safety. However, today's fire took the lives of several fire-fighters and resulted in Mr. C.'s being burned over 30% of his body.

1.   What should nursing care of Mr. C. during the acute phase include?

2.   Mr. C. is going to be transferred to a burn unit. What is a major concern for the nurse?

3.   It is expected that Mr. C. will need an autograft for his facial burns. What assessments and interventions are expected of the nurse for a patient receiving an autograft?

CASE STUDY #2

Mr. G. was golfing during a storm. He attempted to leave the golf course as it started to rain but was struck by lighting as he approached a tree. Mr. G. has a wife and three children.

1.   What are some assessments and interventions for the patient and family dealing with this life-threatening crisis?

2.   If these interventions are successful what outcomes should the nurse expect?

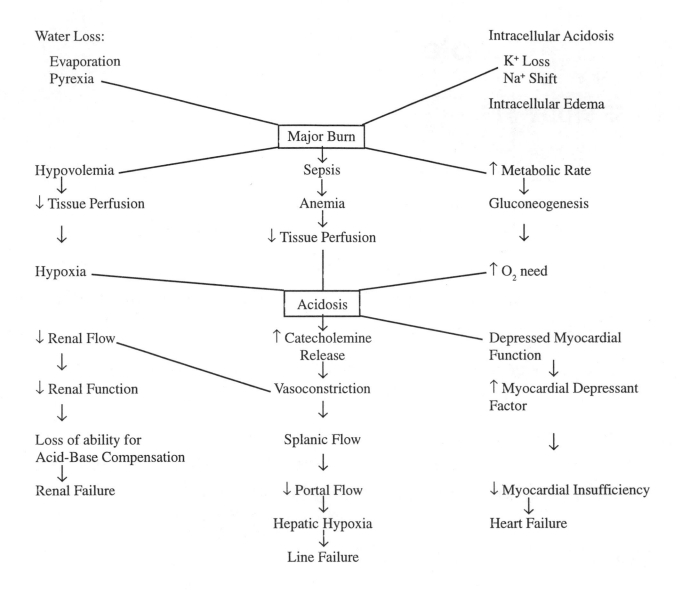

Water Loss:

   Evaporation
   Pyrexia

Intracellular Acidosis

   K^+ Loss
   Na^+ Shift

Intracellular Edema

Major Burn

Hypovolemia → ↓ Tissue Perfusion → ↓ → Hypoxia

Sepsis → Anemia → ↓ Tissue Perfusion

↑ Metabolic Rate → Gluconeogenesis → ↓ → ↑ O_2 need

Acidosis

↓ Renal Flow → ↓ Renal Function → ↓ → Loss of ability for Acid-Base Compensation → Renal Failure

↑ Catecholemine Release → Vasoconstriction → Splanic Flow → ↓ Portal Flow → Hepatic Hypoxia → Line Failure

Depressed Myocardial Function → ↑ Myocardial Depressant Factor → ↓ → ↓ Myocardial Insufficiency → Heart Failure

BURN ESTIMATE AND DIAGRAM

AGE vs. AREA

AREA	Birth 1 yr	1 – 4 yr	5 – 9 yr	10 – 14 yr	15 yr	Adult	2°	3°	Total	Donor Areas
Head	19	17	13	11	9	7				
Neck	2	2	2	2	2	2				
Ant. Trunk	13	13	13	13	13	13				
Post. Trunk	13	13	13	13	13	13				
R. Buttock	2½	2½	2½	2½	2½	2½				
L. Buttock	2½	2½	2½	2½	2½	2½				
Genitalia	1	1	1	1	1	1				
R.U. Arm	4	4	4	4	4	4				
L.U. Arm	4	4	4	4	4	4				
R.L. Arm	3	3	3	3	3	3				
L.L. Arm	3	3	3	3	3	3				
R. Hand	2½	2½	2½	2½	2½	2½				
L. Hand	2½	2½	2½	2½	2½	2½				
R. Thigh	5½	6½	8	8½	9	9½				
L. Thigh	5½	6½	8	8½	9	9½				
R. Leg	5	5	5½	6	6½	7				
L. Leg	5	5	5½	6	6½	7				
R. Foot	3½	3½	3½	3½	3½	3½				
L. Foot	3½	3½	3½	3½	3½	3½				
						TOTAL				

BURN DIAGRAM

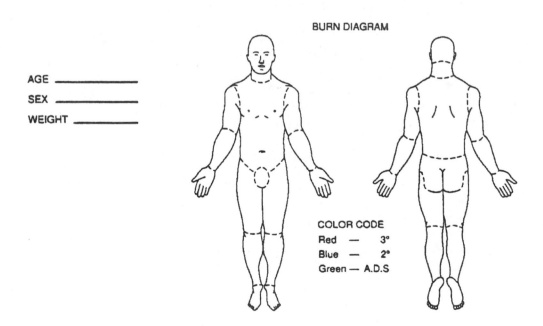

AGE _____

SEX _____

WEIGHT _____

COLOR CODE
Red — 3°
Blue — 2°
Green — A.D.S

Figure 15–7. Burn estimate and diagram. The form depicted was developed and is used by the US Army Institute of Surgical Research. Based on the Lund and Browder chart with Berkow formula, it allows for more accurate assessment of extent of burn injury based on age and depth of injury.

Pathophysiology of Extensive* Burn Injury
(* Injury to > 25% of Total Body Surface Area {TBSA})

LOCAL RESPONSE

Cellular Injury Due to Heat

> Release of cellular enzymes
> Release of vasoactive substances
> Activation of complement

Altered Vascular Membrane Permeability

Shift of protein, fluid and electrolytes   - - - - - -> in cell transmembrane potential due to
at capillary level from intravascular space   fluid and electrolyte shifts ———>Cellular Edema
to extravascular space. (third spacing)   (Restored in 24–36 hours with adequate
($\downarrow$ U.O.; $\uparrow$ HCT; $Na^+ + K^+$ serum imbalances)   fluid resuscitation)

Significant Fluid Resuscitation Required

Volume and Oncotic Pressure Effects

Extensive Edema in Burned and Unburned Areas
(Maximum: 18–24 hours post-burn)

SYSTEMIC RESPONSE

Bi-phasic Hypofunction-Hyperfunction Pattern of All Systems

Maximum Response with 50% TBSA Injury

Normal Organ Function Returns when Wounds Heal or Are Covered

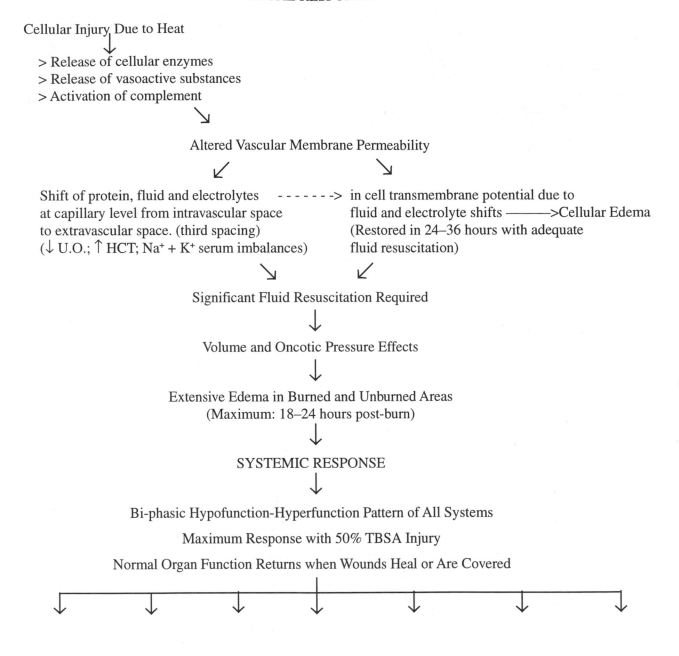

DEPTHS OF BURN INJURY

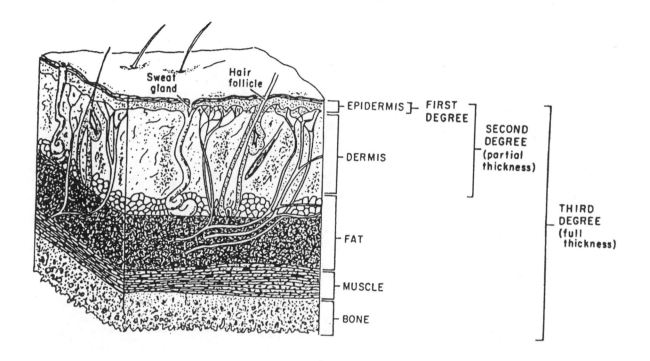

Figure 15–1. Depth of burn injury determines whether a burn will heal or require skin grafting. First- and second-degree burns will heal because they are partial thickness; thus, the elements necessary to generate new skin remain. Full-thickness injury destroys all dermal appendages and requires skin grafting to acheive coverage. (From Kravitz, M.: Thermal Injuries. In: Cardona, V. D., et al: Trauma Nursing: From Resuscitation Through Rehabilitation. Philadelphia, W. B. Saunders, 1988, Fig 28–1, p. 709.)

Major Burn Injury: Primary Survey

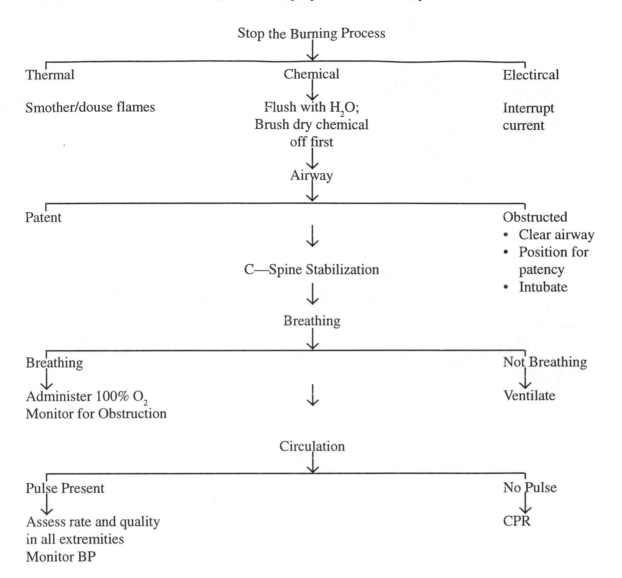

Stop the Burning Process

Thermal	Chemical	Electircal
Smother/douse flames	Flush with H_2O; Brush dry chemical off first	Interrupt current

Airway

Patent		Obstructed
		• Clear airway
		• Position for patency
		• Intubate

C—Spine Stabilization

Breathing

Breathing		Not Breathing
Administer 100% O_2 Monitor for Obstruction		Ventilate

Circulation

Pulse Present		No Pulse
Assess rate and quality in all extremities Monitor BP		CPR

Figure 16–5: Major Burn Injury—Primary Survey

Major Burn Injury: Secondary Survey

Airway
↓
Remains patent and artificial airway is secured

Breathing
↓
Assess ABGs and continue oxygenation as appropriate
Assess need for escharotomy in circumferential burns of chest wall

Circulation
↓
(Pulse Present)

Prevent Shock
- IV access (large bore catheters)
- Assess % Burn—Rule of Nines
- Obtain patient weight
- Calculate fluids:
  2–4 ml LR/Wt in kg/% burn
- Administer fluids:
  ½ 1st 8 hours
  ¼ 2nd 8 hours
  ¼ 3rd 8 hours
- Monitor for adequate urine
  output

Prevent Tissue Damage
- Evaluate pulses in extremities with full-thickness injury circumferentially
- Assess need for escharotomy
- ECG on patients with electric injury

Head-to-Toe Assessments of Other Injuries
↓

Stabilize associated injuries
Tetanus immunization

Past medical history
Referral to burn center

Figure 16–6: Major Burn Injury—Secondary Survey

Glossary

Abandonment   the severance of a professional relationship while a patient is still in need of health care (Chapter 3)

Aberrant conduction   abnormal route by which impulse travels through ventricles (Chapter 4)

Acini cells   pancreatic cells that secrete major pancreatic enzymes such as trypsinogen and chymotrypsinogen (Chapter 14)

ACLS Algorithm   sequence of interventions used to provide advanced cardiac life support (Chapter 7)

Acute   occurs rapidly with little time for compensation (Chapter 11)

Acute renal failure   abrupt cessation of renal function (Chapter 12)

Acute tubular necrosis (ATN)   ischemic injury that extends to basement membrane of nephron (Chapter 8)

Adenosine triphosphate (ATP)   cellular energy (Chapter 12)

Adhesion   attachment of platelets to nonplatelet surfaces (Chapter 13)

Adult respiratory distress syndrome (ARDS)   noncardiogenic pulmonary edema resulting from lung insult (Chapter 11)

Advance directives   a communication that specifies a person's preference regarding medical treatment if he or she should become incapacitated (Chapter 3)

Advanced cardiac life support (ACLS)   standards and guidelines for CPR and emergency cardiac care including airway management and ventilation, IV access, drugs, and treatment of cardiac dysrhythmias (Chapter 7)

Afterload   pressure or resistance to blood flow out of the ventricle (Chapter 5)

Aggregation   adherence of platelets to each other to form plugs (Chapter 13)

Acquired immune deficiency syndrome (AIDS)   syndrome, caused by HIV, resulting in dysfunction of cell-mediated immunity as the virus causes a deficiency in T-helper lymphocyte (Chapter 13)

Albumin   one of a group of simple proteins found in the blood as serum albumin (Chapter 12)

Aluretic   something that promotes excretion of sodium chloride in the urine (Chapter 12)

Alveolar ventilation   amount of gas entering alveoli per minute (Chapter 11)

Ammonia   formed by decomposition of nitrogen-containing substances such as protein (Chapter 12)

Anabolisms   building proteins with positive nitrogen balance (Chapter 14)

Anaerobic metabolism   metabolism without oxygen (Chapter 8)

Anaphylactic shock   antigen initiates antigen-antibody reaction (Chapter 8)

Anemia reduction in number of circulating RBCs or hemoglobin (Chapter 13)

Anger emotional defense to protect individual's integrity (Chapter 2)

Angina chest pain associated with myocardial ischemia (Chapter 9)

Anthropometric pertaining to measuring the human body and its parts (Chapter 12)

Antidysrhythmics drugs that suppress ectopic cardiac activity (Chapters 4 and 9)

Antiemetic an agent that prevents vomiting (Chapter 12)

Anuria urine volume less than 100 ml/24 hr (Chapter 12)

Arterial blood gasses (ABGs) reflect oxygenation, adequacy of gas exchange in lungs, and acid-base status (Chapter 6)

Arteriovenous shunt surgically implanted extracorporeal apparatus used to connect an artery and a vein (Chapter 12)

Arteriovenous fistula internal surgically created communication between an artery and a vein (Chapter 12)

Ascites accumulation of fluid in peritoneum (Chapter 14)

Assist/control (A/C) ventilation ventilator delivers a preset tidal volume whenever patient exerts a negative inspiratory effort (If patient does not spontaneously trigger ventilator, the patient will receive the preset rate.) (Chapter 6)

Asterixis flapping tremor of hand, early sign of hepatic disease (Chapter 14)

Asthma reversible airway obstruction caused by bronchospasm (Chapter 11)

Asynchronous mode pacer does not synchronize its pacemaking with the patient's intrinsic pacemaking (Chapter 4)

Asystole ventricular standstill (Chapter 4)

Atelectasis collapsed alveoli (Chapter 11)

Atheroma atherosclerotic lesion, plaque (Chapter 9)

Atrial kick atrial contraction near the end of diastole adding approximately 30% to ventricular volume (Chapter 4)

Atrioventricular (AV) block impairment in conduction of impulses from atria to ventricles (Chapter 4)

Automatic implantable cardioverter defibrillator (AICD) implanted generator and sensing device that recognizes lethal rhythms and provides an electric shock (Chapter 7)

Automatic external defibrillator (AED) detects ventricular fibrillation and automatically delivers countershock (Chapter 7)

Automaticity ability of the heart cell to beat spontaneously (Chapter 9)

Autonomic dysreflexia exaggerated sympathetic nervous system response to stimuli (e.g., bladder distention, bowel impaction) in spinal cord lesions above T6; medical emergency (Chapter 10)

Autotranfusion patient's own blood is collected, filtered, and reinfused back into the patient (Chapter 9)

AV dissociation complete heart block, no atrial impulses are conducted to ventricles (Chapter 4)

Babinski reflex (UMN lesion/corticospinal) dorsiflexion of great toe and fanning of other toes in response to test (Chapter 10)

Baroreceptors sensitive to stretch and pressure (Chapter 9)

Barotrauma presence of extra alveolar air (Chapter 6)

Basal metabolic rate energy required to perform physiologic processes at rest (Chapter 14)

Basic life support (BLS) one-person CPR (Chapter 7)

Beneficence duty to provide benefits to others (Chapter 3)

Beta blockers drugs that block or diminish the beta effects of the SNS (Chapter 4)

Bilirubin physiologically inactive pigment, metabolic end product of degradation of hemoglobin (Chapter 14)

Biot's respirations   cycles of breaths varying in depth with varying periods of apnea (Chapter 6)

Bipolar   two electrodes encased within pacing catheter (Chapter 4)

Bradycardia   slow heart rate, usually less than 60 beats per minute (Chapter 4)

Bradypnea   respiratory rate less than 10 per minute (Chapter 6)

Brain death   complete and irreversible cessation of brain function occurs (Chapter 3)

Bucking ventilator   patient tries to exhale during inspiratory phase of ventilator (Chapter 11)

Buffer system   mechanism for neutralizing acids (Chapter 6)

Burnout   syndrome of emotional exhaustion, depersonalization, and reduced personal accomplishment (Chapter 2)

Calcium channel blockers   block some of calcium's movement across cardiac cell membrane, which slows the rate of depolarization (Chapter 4)

Calibration   operation performed to ensure numerical accuracy within electrical system (Chapter 5)

Capillary refill   gross estimate of perfusion, measured from when patient's nail pales after it is depressed until it becomes pink again, usually 1 to 2 seconds (Chapter 8)

Capture   chamber depolarization initiated by pacemaker (Chapter 4)

Cardiac index (CI)   measured in liters/minute/ square meter, takes into account patient body surface area (normal CI: 2.5 to 4/min/m^2) (Chapter 5)

Cardiac glycosides   drugs that increase strength of contraction, suppress sinus depolarization and atrial irritability, and slow conduction through AV node (Chapter 4)

Cardiac reserve   capacity of the heart to adjust to increased demands (Chapter 9)

Cardiac output (CO)   flow from heart measured in liters/minute, heart rate (HR) × stroke volume (SV) = cardiac output (CO) (Chapter 5)

Cardiogenic shock   failure of heart to act as an effective pump (Chapter 8)

Cardioversion   delivery of countershock that is synchronized with the patient's cardiac rhythm (Chapter 7)

Catabolism   destructive phase of metabolism, the opposite of anabolism (Chapter 12); breakdown of proteins, negative nitrogen balance (Chapter 14)

Catecholamines   epinephrine and norepinephrine released with sympathetic stimulation (Chapter 8)

Central venous pressure (CVP)   right atrial pressure (Chapter 5)

Chemoreceptors   sensitive to changes in PO_2, PCO_2, and pH_4 blood levels (Chapter 9)

Chemotaxis   movement of additional white blood cells to area of inflammation in response to release of chemical mediators (Chapter 12)

Cheyne-Stokes respiration   deep respirations that become increasingly shallow followed by a period of apnea (Chapters 6 and 10)

Chronic   develops over time, compensatory defenses active (Chapter 11)

Chronic bronchitis   productive cough for at least three consecutive months for at least two consecutive years (Chapter 11)

Chronic obstructive pulmonary disease (COPD)   group of disorders that results in obstruction of airflow in the lungs (Chapter 11)

Chronotropism   heart rate (Chapter 8)

Chvostek's sign   spasm of facial muscles after tapping the side of the face over the area of the facial nerve (Chapter 12); Chvostek's sign (hypocalcemia)—tap face over facial nerve causing spasm of lip, nose, or face, increase in neuromuscular excitability (Chapter 14)

Chyme   semifluid mixture of food with gastric secretions (Chapter 14)

Circadian rhythm   biological rhythms occurring in 24-hour cycles (Chapter 2)

Coagulopathy   defect in blood clotting mechanism (Chapter 12)

Code/arrest emergency situation requiring life-saving resuscitation and interventions (Chapter 7)

Colloid solution containing molecules that increase osmotic pressure within the vascular space (Chapter 8)

Compliance measure of distensibility of lung and chest wall (Chapter 6)

Computed tomography (CT) scan noninvasive radiographic technique that produces a precise reconstructed image of structures (Chapter 12)

Conductivity heart's ability to transmit electrical impulses rapidly and efficiently to all areas of heart (Chapter 9)

Congestive heart failure (CHF) clinical state in which heart is unable to maintain cardiac output to meet body's metabolic demands (Chapter 9)

Conjugated/direct bilirubin bound with either glucuronic acid or glucuronic sulfate so that it becomes soluble in bile (Chapter 14)

Continuous positive airway pressure (CPAP) augments functional residual capacity during spontaneous breaths (Chapter 6)

Contractility intrinsic ability of muscle fibers to shorten (Chapter 5)

Controlled mechanical ventilation (CMV) ventilator delivers a preset tidal volume at a preset rate regardless of patient's respiratory effort (Chapter 6)

Coronary artery bypass graft (CABG) surgical procedure in which ischemic myocardium is revascularized (Chapter 9)

Coronary artery disease (CAD)/Arteriosclerotic heart disease (ASHD) partial or total occlusion of the coronary arteries by atherosclerosis (Chapter 9)

Crackles short, explosive, nonmusical, and discontinuous sounds indicating presence of fluid in alveoli and airways (Chapter 6)

Crash cart cart containing basic emergency equipment and medications (Chapter 7)

Creatinine metabolic by-product of muscle (Chapter 12)

Creatinine clearance estimate of glomerular filtration rate measured in ml/min., normal: 120 ml/min. (Chapter 12)

Crystalloid electrolyte solutions that move freely from intravascular space into the tissues (Chapter 8)

Cyanosis bluish tint to skin because of circulating deoxygenated hemoglobin (Chapter 8)

Damped waveform pressure waveform decreased in amplitude indicative of interference with impulse transmission (Chapter 5)

Dead space areas of airway that do not exchange gases (Chapter 11)

Decerebrate abnormal posturing with extension of all extremities and clenched jaws (Pons/midbrain) (Chapter 10)

Decorticate abnormal posturing with flexed upper extremities and extended lower extremities (cortical/subcortical/diencephalon) (Chapter 10)

Deep vein thrombosis (DVT) thrombophlebitis of deep veins of calf (Chapter 11)

Defibrillation delivery of an electrical current to the heart using a defibrillator, completely depolarizes the heart and disrupts the impulses causing the dysrhythmia (Chapter 7)

Demand mode pacemaker generates an impulse only when the patient cannot generate his or her own (Chapter 4)

Depolarization active phase of electrical activity (Chapter 4)

Desynchronization refers to disruption in patterns (Chapter 2)

Diabetes insipidus deficiency of ADH resulting in excretion of excessive dilute urine (Chapter 12)

Dialysate fluid used to remove or deliver compounds or electrolytes that the failing kidney cannot produce or excrete properly (Chapter 12)

Dialysis separation of solutes by differential diffusion through a porous membrane between two solutions (Chapter 12)

Diastole muscle resting, uncontracted state (Chapter 4)

Dicrotic notch   small notch on downstroke of arterial waveform resulting from closure of aortic valve (Chapter 5)

Diffusion   movement across semipermeable membrane from area of high concentration to area of lower concentration (Chapters 6 and 12)

Diffusion defect   changes in distance between alveoli and pulmonary capillary (Chapter 11)

Digestion   breakdown of nutrients for absorption (Chapter 14)

Disequilibrium syndrome   cerebral edema resulting from rapid, large decreases in serum BUN and creatinine, occurs usually after one to three dialysis treatments (Chapter 12)

Disseminated intravascular coagulation (DIC)   coagulation in microcirculation and paradoxical hemorrhage (Chapter 8)

Distributive shock   widespread vasodilatation with a decrease in peripheral vascular resistance (Chapter 8)

Doctrine of informed consent   competent adults have a right to self-determination to accept or reject medical or nursing treatment (Chapter 3)

Dromotropy   used to describe speed of conduction (Chapter 4)

Dry body weight   weight below which signs and symptoms of hypotension occur (Chapter 12)

Dyspnea   difficulty breathing (Chapter 11)

Dysrhythmia   abnormal cardiac rhythms (Chapter 4)

Ecchymosis   extravasation of blood into the skin or mucous membrane (Chapter 12)

Ectopic   out of the normal place (Chapter 4)

Ejection fraction   volume of blood ejected during ventricular systole (Chapter 5)

Electrocardiography   process creating a visual tracing of the electrical activity of the cells in the heart (Chapter 4)

Electrophysiology   study of myocardial electrical conduction (Chapter 4)

Embolus   mass undissolved matter floating in blood vessel (Chapter 5)

Emphysema   nonreversible obstructive disease characterized by destruction of alveolar walls and connective tissue (Chapter 11)

Encephalopathy   alteration in brain functions due to ammonia toxicity or other metabolite derangements (Chapter 14)

End-tidal carbon dioxide (etCO$_2$)   capnometry, measurement of expired CO$_2$ that correlates with PaCO$_2$ (Chapter 6)

Endocardium   inner endothelial layer of heart (Chapter 9)

Endocrine   secrete internally (Chapter 14)

Endotracheal tube (ETT)   artificial airway inserted into the trachea through either the mouth or nose (Chapter 6)

Epicardium   outer layer of heart muscle (Chapter 9)

Erythrocyte   red blood cell (Chapter 5)

Erythropoietin   hormone produced by the kidneys that stimulates formation and differentiation of red blood cells (Chapters 12 and 13)

Exacerbate   worsen (Chapter 2)

Excitability   cell's ability to respond to electrochemical stimulation (Chapter 9)

Exocrine   secrete through a duct externally (Chapter 14)

External pacer/transcutaneous pacer (TCP)   cardiac pacer that works through the chest wall (Chapter 7)

Extracorporeal   outside the body (Chapter 12)

Fibrillation   erratic impulse formation (Chapter 4)

Fibrinogen   blood protein that participates in coagulation (Chapter 13)

Fibrinolysis   fibrinogen and fibrin digested via plasmin (Chapter 13)

Filtration   movement of fluid across a semipermeable membrane from an area of great pressure to an area of lesser pressure (Chapter 12)

Fluid challenge   volume of fluid given over specified time (e.g., 10 ml/min. over 10 min.) to assess patient's hemodynamic response to rapid administration of fluid (Chapter 8)

Fraction of inspired oxygen (FiO$_2$) amount of O$_2$ delivered (Chapter 6)

Gastric lavage instill fluid and remove intermittently via NG tube to asses bleeding and cleanse the stomach (Chapter 14)

Gastric mucosal barrier physiologic barrier impermeable to hydrochloric acid (Chapter 14)

Glomerular filtration filtration of fluid via the glomerular sieve into Bowman's capsule (Chapter 12)

Gluconeogenesis making glucose from proteins and fats (Chapter 14)

Glycogenesis storing glycogen (Chapter 14)

Glycogenolysis forming glucose by splitting glycogen stored in the liver (Chapter 14)

Guaiac solution used in testing for occult blood in the feces (Chapter 12)

Gut intestines (Chapter 14)

Haustrations contractile activity of colon (Chapter 14)

HCO$_3$ concentration of sodium bicarbonate in the blood (22 to 26 mEq/L) (Chapter 6)

Hematemesis bloody vomitus (Chapter 14)

Hematochezia bright red blood from rectum (Chapter 14)

Hematopoiesis formation and development of blood cells (Chapter 13)

Hematuria blood in urine (Chapter 12)

Hemodialysis extracorporeal separation of solutes by differential diffusion through a celluloid membrane (Chapter 12)

Hemodilution increase in volume blood plasma resulting in reduced relative concentration of RBCs (Chapter 8)

Hemodynamics interrelationship of various physical forces that affect the blood's circulation through body (Chapter 5)

Hemofiltration/Continuous arterial venous hemofiltration (CAVH) convective mode of blood cleansing that is controlled by the patient's hydrostatic pressure (Chapter 12)

Hemoptysis bloody productive cough (Chapter 11)

Herniation syndromes a portion of brain tissue is pushed through available openings in the cranial cavity (e.g., CN and BV openings, foramen magnum, tentorial notch) (Chapter 10)

HHNC hyperosmolar state, less formation ketones that DKA, resulting in volume depletion (Chapter 14)

Histamine two types: H$_1$ receptors that mediate smooth muscle contraction and capillary dilation and H$_2$ that mediate acceleration of heart rate and increase gastric acid secretion (Chapter 14)

Hunger intrinsic desire for food (Chapter 14)

Hydrostatic pushing pressure with blood vessel (Chapter 8)

Hypercapnia excessive CO$_2$ (Chapter 11)

Hyperglycemia

Hyperinflation delivery of breaths 1 to 1.5 times tidal volume (Chapter 6)

Hyperlipidemia high levels lipids in the blood (Chapter 9)

Hyperosmolar solution contains all known essential nutrients (Chapter 14)

Hyperoxygenation delivery of 100% O$_2$ (Chapter 6)

Hyperventilation three to five quick breaths (Chapter 6)

Hypocarbia low CO$_2$ (Chapter 11)

Hypoglycemic body not receiving normal glucose (Chapter 14)

Hypovolemic shock inadequate circulating blood volume to fill vascular space (Chapter 8)

Hypoxemia low O$_2$ in the blood (Chapter 11)

Hypoxia low O$_2$ in tissues (Chapter 11)

ICU syndrome usually occurs after 48 hours with symptoms range from perceptual distortion to vivid hallucinations (Chapter 2)

Idioventricular rhythm escape rhythm generated by the Purkinje fibers (Chapter 4)

Immunity the body's ability to resist and fight infection (Chapter 13)

Increased intracranial pressure (IICP) pressure over 15 mmHg within the cranial cavity due to increased volume from increased blood flow or increased bulk of brain tissue (Chapter 10)

Infective endocarditis infection of endocardial tissue (Chapter 9)

Infradian rhythms exist longer than 24 hours (Chapter 2)

Insufficiency valve leaflets do not approximate (Chapter 9)

Integument the skin (Chapter 12)

Intercostal between the ribs (Chapter 4)

Intermittent mandatory ventilation (IMV)/ Synchronized intermittent mandatory ventilation (SIMV) delivers a preset volume at a preset rate and allows patient to breathe spontaneously between ventilator breaths (Chapter 6)

Intra-aortic balloon pump (IABP) counterpulsation device that increases coronary perfusion without increasing myocardial work (Chapter 8)

Intra-arterial monitoring invasive technique of monitoring arterial blood pressure (Chapter 5)

Intrapulmonary shunting blood shunted past lung and returned to left heart unoxygenated (Chapter 11)

Intravenous pyelography (IVP) IV contrast medium to visualize kidneys, ureters, and bladder (Chapter 12)

Intrinsic factor necessary for absorption of Vitamin B_{12} (Chapter 14)

Irreversible coma/Persistent vegetative state some brain function remains intact (Chapter 3)

Islets of Langerhans alpha and beta cells that perform endocrine functions of pancreas (Chapter 14)

Joules/Watt-seconds energy delivered by defibrillator (Chapter 7)

Junctional/Nodal rhythm rhythm generated by AV node or junctional tissue (Chapter 4)

Ketoacidosis acute state, dehydration, elevated glucose levels, excessive formation of ketones (Chapter 14)

Ketonia excess of ketones (Chapter 14)

Korotkoff's sounds vibrations of arterial wall (Chapter 5)

Kupffer's cells phagocytic cells of liver (Chapter 14)

Kussmaul's respiration deep, regular, rapid respirations (Chapter 6)

Left atrial pressure reflection left ventricular preload (Chapter 5)

Leukocyte white blood cell (Chapter 5)

Leukopenia deficiency of white blood cells (Chapter 8)

Lipolysis splitting of fat cells (Chapter 14)

Manual resuscitation bag (MRB) device used to ventilate and oxygenate a patient who is not breathing (Chapter 6)

Mastication act of chewing (Chapter 14)

Mean arterial pressure (MAP) normal: 70 to 100 mmHg (Chapter 5)

$$\frac{SBP + (2 \times DBP)}{3} = MAP$$

Mechanical ventilation supportive therapy to maintain normal gas exchange in patients with respiratory failure (Chapter 6)

Melena shiny, black, foul-smelling stool resulting from degradation of blood (Chapter 14)

Metabolic alkalosis too much HCO_3 (Chapter 6)

Metabolic acidosis too little HCO_3 (Chapter 6)

Microcirculation portion of vascular bed between arterioles and venules where exchange occurs between blood and cells (Chapter 8)

Micturition urination (Chapter 12)

Military antishock trousers (MAST) increase peripheral vascular resistance, stop-gap measure only (Chapter 8)

Milliamperes (MA) electrical output of pacer (Chapter 4)

Minute ventilation volume of air breathed in a minute (Chapter 6)

Mixed venous oxygen saturation (SVO$_2$) oxygen saturation of blood in pulmonary artery, helps evaluate oxygen supply and demand, normal: 60% to 80% (Chapter 5)

Multifocal multiple sites generating impulses (Chapter 4)

Multiple organ failure (MOF) more than one organ unable to maintain its own function (Chapter 8)

Murmur sound caused by a turbulence of blood flow through the valves (Chapter 9)

Myocardial infarction (MI) death of myocardial tissue due to lack of blood supply (Chapter 9)

Myocardium middle muscular layer of heart (Chapter 9)

Nasopharyngeal airway soft rubber or latex tube inserted into nares and nasopharynx to help maintain an open airway (Chapter 6)

Negative feedback

Negligence failure to act in a reasonable and prudent manner, acts of commission: giving wrong medication, acts of omission: failing to raise side rails (Chapter 3)

Nephrosonography high frequency sound waves reflect off kidneys and are transformed into an image (Chapter 12)

Neurogenic shock disturbance in nervous system that affects vasomotor center (Chapter 8)

Neuromuscular blocking agent drug that paralyzes skeletal muscles (Chapter 11)

Nitrates vasodilator used to relieve or prevent chest pain and lower blood pressure (Chapter 9)

Nocturia voiding during the night (Chapter 12)

Nonmaleficence explicit duty to not intentionally harm others (Chapter 3)

Oliguria urine volume of 100 to 400 ml/24 hr (Chapter 12)

Opsonization antibody and complement attach to phagocytic cells (Chapter 13)

Oral airway rigid tube that prevents tongue from falling into pharynx (Chapter 6)

Oscilloscope a screen to display pressure waveforms (Chapter 5)

Osmosis movement water across a semipermeable membrane from an area of lesser concentration to an area of greater concentration (Chapter 12)

Osmotic pressure pulling pressure exerted by proteins within vascular space (Chapter 8)

Oxygen saturation (SaO$_2$) amount of oxygen bound to hemoglobin: 93% to 99% (Chapter 6)

Oxyhemoglobin dissociation curve relationship between PaO$_2$ and SaO$_2$ (Chapter 6)

P wave atrial depolarization (Chapter 4)

Pacemaker device that delivers electrical energy to pace the heart (Chapter 4)

Palpitations irregular heart beat (Chapter 9)

Pancreatic alpha cells secrete glucagon (Chapter 14)

Pancreatic beta cells secrete insulin (Chapter 14)

Paradoxical pulse exaggerated fluctuation of arterial pressure during respiratory cycle (Chapter 7)

Parasympathetic nervous system (PNS) cranial sacral segment of autonomic nervous system/cholinergic (Postganglionid nerve endings go to heart smooth muscle and the glands of the head/neck/thorax/abdominal and pelvic viscera; responses include increase gland secretions of enzymes, pupil constriction, increased peristalsis, decreased heart rate.) (Chapters 4, 10, and 14)

Parenchymal renal failure acute renal failure produced by conditions acting directly on kidney tissue (Chapter 12)

Paroxysmal occurring without warning (Chapter 4)

Partial pressure of oxygen (PaO$_2$) oxygen dissolved in arterial blood: 80 to 100 mmHg (Chapter 6)

Partial pressure of carbon dioxide (PaCO$_2$) carbon dioxide dissolved in arterial plasma: 35 to 45 mmHg (Chapter 6)

Patient Self Determination Act (PSDA) federal law mandating enabling patients to make informed decisions about medical care in advance of terminal medical illness (Chapter 7)

Peak inspiratory pressure peak airway pressure during normal ventilation (Chapter 6)

Percutaneous transluminal coronary angioplasty (PTCA) interventional radiology performed to compress intracoronary lesions to increase blood flow to myocardium (Chapter 9)

Perfusion transportation (Chapter 6)

Pericardiocentesis surgical puncture of percardial sac to remove fluid (Chapter 7)

Pericarditis inflammation of the pericardium (Chapter 12)

Pericardial tamponade accumulation of fluid in pericardial sac that interferes with cardiac filling and emptying (Chapter 7)

Peristalsis movement that propels contents through alimentary canal (Chapter 4)

Peritoneal lavage washing out peritoneal cavity (Chapter 8); instilling fluid into cavity for removal of waste products or toxins (Chapter 14)

Peritoneal dialysis separation of solutes by differential diffusion through the peritoneal membrane, dialysate is instilled in peritoneal cavity (Chapter 12)

Petechiae small purplish hemorrhagic spots on the skin (Chapter 12)

pH concentration of H+ in blood: 7.35 to 7.45   (Chapter 6)

Phagocytosis process by which antigens and damaged cells removed from the tissues (Chapters 12 and 13)

Phlebostatic axis level of the right atrium; fourth intercostal space, midaxillary line (Chapter 5)

Physical stress events or stimuli that alter homeostasis (Chapter 2)

Plasma expander synthetic colloid, high molecular weight solutions to increase blood volume (Chapter 8)

Pleural space area between parietal and visceral pleurae (Chapter 6)

Pleural friction rub getting sound occurring in presence of inflamed pleura (Chapter 6)

Pneumoconstriction airways constrict (Chapter 11)

Pneumothorax air in pleural space (Chapter 6)

Polyuria urine volume in excess of 400 ml/24 hr (Chapter 12)

Positive feedback

Positive pressure ventilation forces air into the lungs via positive pressure (Chapters 6 and 10)

Positive inotrope agent that strengthens myocardial contraction (Chapter 8)

Positive end expiratory pressure (PEEP) pressure applied at end of expiration that keeps small airways open so gas exchange occurs at alveolar level, which can lead to complication of increased intrathoracic pressure and thus decreased venous return, deceased right ventricular filling, and decreased cardiac output (Chapters 6 and 10)

Postrenal failure acute renal failure as a result of obstruction to flow of urine (Chapter 12)

Powerlessness perceived lack of control (Chapter 2)

Preload left ventricular end diastolic volume (LVEDV) (Chapter 5)

Prerenal failure acute renal failure caused by interference with renal perfusion (Chapter 12)

Pressure-cycled ventilator air flows into lungs until a preset pressure is reached (Chapter 6)

Pressure support ventilation (PSV) preset level of positive pressure used to assist spontaneously breathing patient (Chapter 6)

Prodromal pertaining to initial stage of disease (Chapter 8)

Pruritus severe itching (Chapter 12)

Psychological stress events real or imagined that are perceived to result in danger (Chapter 2)

Pulmonary artery catheter multilumen balloon-tipped flow-directed catheter having capabilities to measure CVP, PAP, and CO; may also measure SVO_2 and/or have transvenous pacing capability (Chapter 5)

Pulmonary artery wedge pressure (PAWP)/ Pulmonary capillary wedge pressure (PCWP) mean pressure of 6 to 12 mmHg reflecting left ventricular function (Chapter 5)

Pulmonary edema acute life-threatening form of CHF (Chapter 9)

Pulmonary artery pressure (PAP) pressure in pulmonary artery, norm approximately 25/10 mmHg (Chapter 5)

Pulmonary embolus (PE) blockage of pulmonary artery from a thrombus that usually arises from systemic veins and results in obstruction of blood flow to lung tissue (Chapter 11)

Pulmonary toilet pulmonary hygiene, airway clearance, and so on (Chapter 11)

Pulse oximetry (SpO_2) reflects SaO_2 via a sensor on finger, forehead, ear, or toe (Chapter 6)

Pulse pressure difference between SBP and DBP (Chapter 5)

Purpura condition characterized by hemorrhages into the skin, mucous membranes, and internal organs (Chapter 12)

QRS complex ventricular depolarization (Chapter 4)

Renal angiography contrast material injected into renal arteries via catheter placed in aorta to visualize renal blood flow and vessels (Chapter 12)

Renal osteodystrophy generalized pathological changes in the bone associated with renal failure (Chapter 12)

Renin enzyme produced by the kidneys that acts on angiotensin (Chapter 12)

Repolarization resting phase during which electrical activity is minimal (Chapter 4)

Respiratory acidosis too much CO_2 (Chapter 6)

Respiratory alkalosis too little CO_2 (Chapter 6)

Respiratory failure impaired O_2 uptake and/or CO_2 elimination (Chapter 11)

Rhythmicity ability heart muscle to depolarize rhythmically (Chapter 9)

S_1 first heart sound ("lubb") caused by closure of mitral and tricuspid valves (Chapter 9)

S_2 second heart sound ("dup") caused by closure aortic and pulmonic valves (Chapter 9)

S_3 caused by rapid blood flow into a nonpliable ventricle (Chapter 9)

S_4 caused by atrial contraction that is more forceful than normal (Chapter 9)

Sclerotherapy injecting sclerosing solutions into vessels (Chapter 14)

Sense (sensitivity) pacer's ability to "see" the patient's intrinsic heart beat (Chapter 4)

Sensory overload two or more stimuli confronting patient at a greater level than normal (Chapter 2)

Sensory deprivation decrease in amount of meaningful sensory input (Chapter 2)

Septic shock overwhelming systemic infection (Chapter 8)

Shock clinical syndrome characterized by inadequate tissue perfusion that results in impaired cellular metabolism (Chapter 8)

SIADH inappropriate release or secretion of ADH (vasopressin), resulting in improper function of feedback mechanism; water is retained, leading to dilutional hyponatremia and increased extracellular fluid volume (Chapter 14)

Sigh breath that is 1.5 to 2 times tidal volume (Chapter 6)

Sinus rhythm optimal cardiac rhythm, sinus node generates an electrical impulse that is conducted down the normal conduction pathway depolarizing all cardiac cells (Chapter 4)

Splanchnic circulation blood supply to organs within the abdomen (Chapter 14)

Stomatitis inflammation of the mouth (Chapter 12)

Stroke volume amount of blood ejected with each ventricular contraction (Chapter 9)

Subcutaneous emphysema air beneath the skin's surface (Chapter 6)

Subendocardial MI involves a partial thickness of the inner half of heart muscle (Chapter 9)

Superficial partial thickness injury involves epidermis (first degree) or variable portions of the dermis (second degree); deep partial thickness involves injury of epidermis, most of dermis; full thickness injury is destruction of all layers of the skin down to or past subcutaneous fat, fascia, muscles, and /or bone, including nerves (Chapter 16)

Suppuration pus formed via phagocytosis (Chapter 13)

Surfactant substance produced in alveolar wall that decreases alveolar surface tension (Chapter 11)

Sympathetic nervous system thoracolumbar part of autonomic nervous system/adrenergic (Post ganglionic fibers go to heart, smooth muscle, and glands of entire body; response to catecholamine release includes pupil dilation, increased heart rate, and bronchial dilation.) (Chapter 10)

Synchronizers things that occur at same time (Chapter 2)

Syncope transient loss of consciousness due to inadequate blood flow to brain (Chapter 12)

Systemic vascular resistance (SVR) afterload (Chapter 8)

Systole contraction of cardiac muscle (Chapter 4)

T wave ventricular repolarization (Chapter 4)

Tachycardia fast heart rate, usually greater than 100 (Chapter 4)

Tachypnea respiratory rate greater than 20 (Chapter 6)

Tension pneumothorax air enters pleural space, cannot escape, pressure increases, lung may collapse (Chapter 7)

Thermodilution method measuring CO by injecting a known amount of solution at a known temperature into the right atrium and then measuring the resulting drop in temperature downstream in the pulmonary artery (Chapter 5)

Third spacing fluid accumulating in areas outside the blood vessels reduces intravascular volume (Chapter 8)

Threshold minimum amount of electrical energy required to achieve capture (Chapter 4)

Thrombocytopenia deficiency of platelets (Chapter 13)

Thrombolytic agent that destroys clots (Chapter 8)

Thrombopoietin regulates production and maturation of platelets (Chapter 13)

Thrombosis blood clot (Chapter 5)

Tidal volume volume of normal breath, 10 to 15 ml/kg (Chapter 6)

Time-cycled ventilator air flows into lungs until a preset amount of time has elapsed (Chapter 6)

Total parenteral nutrition (TPN) (Chapter 14)

Tracheostomy tube artificial airway inserted via a surgically created opening in the trachea (Chapter 6)

Transducer instrument used to sense physiologic events and transform them into electric signals (Chapter 5)

Transferrin globulin in the blood that binds and transports iron (Chapter 12)

Transmural MI involves the entire thickness of the heart muscle (Chapter 9)

Transthoracic through the chest wall (thorax) (Chapter 4)

Transvenous through the vein (Chapter 4)

Trendelenburg's position head down, legs raised (Chapter 5)

Trousseau's sign spasmodic muscular contractions produced by pressure applied to vessels and nerves of the upper arm (Chapter 12); (hypocalcemia)—inflate blood pressure cuff for 1 to 5 minutes occluding circulation of hand causing contraction of fingers and hands, indicates presence of tetany (Chapter 14)

Ultradian rhythms rhythms that exist less than 24 hours (Chapter 2)

Ultrafiltration removal of plasma, water, and some smaller molecular weight particles using an osmotic gradient (Chapter 12)

Unconjugated/indirect bilirubin free, insoluble in plasma, carried in blood attached to albumin reflective of prehepatic problems (e.g., increased red blood cell production) or problems with ability to conjugate in the liver (Chapter 14)

Urea formed from ammonia in the liver, final product of protein metabolism in body (Chapter 12)

Uremia toxic conditions produced by retention of nitrogenous substances normally excreted by kidneys (Chapter 12)

Uremic encephalopathy dysfunction of the brain as a result of uremia (Chapter 12)

Uremic frost uremic waste crystallizing on skin from severe azotemia (Chapter 12)

Uremic halitosis offensive breath from uremia (Chapter 12)

Urochrome pigment that makes urine yellow (Chapter 12)

Vagal maneuvers used to stimulate vagus nerve to slow heart rate (Chapter 4)

Vagolytic drug that blocks effects of vagus nerve and increase heart rate (Chapters 4 and 8)

Valsalva's maneuver forcible exhalation against closed glottis, which results in increased intrathoracic pressure and vagal stimulation (Chapter 10)

Vascular resistance opposition blood flow exerted by blood vessels (Chapter 5)

Vasoactive drugs drugs which alter lumen size of blood vessels (Chapter 5)

Vasodilators drugs to relax smooth muscle in arteries, arterioles, or veins (Chapter 9)

Vasopressor agent that causes vasoconstriction (Chapter 8)

Ventilation transport of air in and out of alveoli (Chapter 6)

Ventilation-perfusion mismatching ratio between ventilation and perfusion (Chapter 11)

Viscera internal organs, especially abdominal organs (Chapter 12)

Vital capacity maximum volume of gas that can be forcefully exhaled after maximum inspiration (Chapter 6)

Vitamin K factors II (prothrombin), VII, IX, and X (Chapter 14)

Volume-cycled ventilator air flows into lungs until a present volume has been reached (Chapter 6)

Water manometer fluid filled tube that measures CVP (Chapter 5)

Weaning process of removing a patient from mechanical ventilation (Chapter 6)

Wheezes continuous sounds resulting from air passing through narrow passages (Chapter 6)

Zero referencing operation performed to eliminate influence of atmospheric pressure (Chapter 5)

Sources

Myocardial Infarction (3) and CHF (4). *Medical/Surgical Nursing.* (1994). Two videos, 30 minutes each. Mosby.

Lukas, Jami. (1996). *Clinical Management of Heart Failure.* Three videos, 480 minutes. Arlington Heights: Northwest Community Healthcare.

Management of End Stage Heart Failure. (1996). Video, 55 minutes. AHA/Westcott Communications.

Heart Failure Mechanisms and Medical Therapies. (1996). Video, 90 minutes. AHA/Westcott Communications.

Congestive Heart Failure: Triple Drug Therapy for Prevention and Management. (1993). Video. Richmond: Virginia Commonwealth University.

Anatomy of Congestive Heart Failure. (1991). Roche Laboratories.

Marks, Kathy. *Congestive Heart Failure.* (1995). Video, 30 minutes. Augusta: Medical College of Georgia.

Management of Heart Failure. (1995). Video, 60 minutes. Network for Continuing Medical Education.

Wolfe, Massie, Brindis. *Management of CHF.* (1993). Video, 49 minutes. Kaiser Foundation Health Plan.

Inherited Cardiomyopathies. (1994). Video, 56 minutes. St. Louis: Medical Video Productions.

Prevention of Ventricular Enlargement and Heart Failure following Myocardial Infarction. (1992). Video, 49 minutes. Kluwer Academic Publishers.

Prevention and management of Heart Failure: Value of triple drug therapy. (1993) Video, 57 minutes. Virginia Commonwealth.

Problem Cases in Interventional Cardiology, Part 1. (1994). Video, 14 minutes. St. Louis: Medical Video Productions.

Advances in ACE Inhibition. (1992). Video, 46 minutes. Houston: American Medical Communications: Methodist Hospital System.

Cardiovascular System. (1991). Eight videos, 276 minutes. West Lafayette: Purdue University School of Pharmacy.

Resuscitation Adjuncts and Automated External Defibrillation. (1991). Video, book, four computer disks, and two sound cassettes. Pittsburgh: Actronics.

Attenuation Cardiac Remodeling. (1991). Video, 11 minutes. St. Louis: Medical Video Productions.

Living Well with Coronary Artery Disease. (1995). Video, 38 minutes. Beaverton: Mosby Great Performance, Inc.

Koop, Everett. *Coronary Artery Disease.* (1996). Video, 30 minutes. Time Life Medical.

Diagnosis and Treatment of Coronary Artery Disease. (1994). Video, 30 minutes. Calhoun: NIMCO.

Multivessel Angioplasty in CAD. (1994). Video, 50 minutes. Atlanta: University of Atlanta.

Treatment choices for Ischemic Heart Disease. (1995). Video, 55 minutes. Hanover: Foundation for Informed Medical Decision Making.

The Operation: Coronary Bypass Surgery. (1994). Video, 45 minutes. Princeton: Films for Humanities and Sciences.

Learning EKG Series. (1994). Ten videos, 20 minutes each. Mosby Year Book.

Challenges in Echocardiography: Difficult case presentations and analysis. (1993). Video, 5 minutes.

Coronary Artery Disease. (1991). Video, 30 minutes. New Orleans: Hotel Dieu Hospital.

Noninvasive Assessment of Coronary Anatomy and Physiology: The transesophageal approach. (1991). Video, 17 minutes. St. Louis: Medical Video Productions.

Noninvasive Techniques in Treatment of Coronary Artery Disease. (1991) Video, 21 minutes. St. Louis: Medical Video Productions.

Early Symptoms and Recognition of a Heart Attack. (1995). Video, 46 minutes. Baltimore: St. Agnes Hospital.

Twelve Lead EKG. (1995). Two videos, 3 hours. Staten Island: Education Enterprises.

Adult Acute MI (Advanced Life Support Series). (1994). Video, 14 minutes. Mosby Lifeline Distribution.

GUSTO-1 The Heart of the Matter. (1994). Video, 23 minutes. Westbrough: ASTRA.

Acute Intervention in Management of Myocardial Infarction. (1992). Video, 39 minutes. Marshfield Video Network.

Brown, K. R., et al. *Mastering Dysrhythmias: A problem-solving guide.* (1988)

Brown, K. R., et al. *Mastering Dysrhythmias: A problem-solving guide.* (1988) ECG slide set, 297 slides.

Moorhouse, M. F., et al. *Critical Care Plans: Guidelines for advanced medical-surgical care.* (1987)

Franki, W. S., et al. *Valvular Heart Disease: Comprehensive Evaluation and Treatment.* (2nd ed.) (1993).

Spittell, J. A., Jr. *Contemporary Issues in Peripheral Vascular Disease.* (1992).

Greenspoon, A. J., et al. *Contemporary Management of Ventricular Arrhythmias.* (1992).

Waters, D. D., et al. *Care of the Patient with Previous Coronary Bypass Surgery.* (1991).

Iskandrian, A. S., et al. *Nuclear Cardiac Imaging: Principles and applications.* (2nd ed.) (1995).

Wagner, G. S., et al. *Cardiac Arrhythmias: A practical guide for the clinician.* (2nd ed.) (1994).

Yang, S. S., et al. *From Cardiac Catheterization Data to Hemodynamic Parameters.* (3rd ed.) (1988).

Holmes. D. R., et al. *Interventional Cardiology.* (1989).

Goldberg, X. L., et al. *Exercise for Prevention and Treatment of Illness.* (1994).